BEST OF
999 Reasons to Laugh at I

By Infertile Naomi

Based on the popular blog, '999 Reasons to Laugh at Infertility,' because crying every time you get your period doesn't seem to help.

Check out the blog at www.999reasonstolaugh.com

This book is dedicated to all the future parents who are waiting for their babies. Keep persevering because one day, it will be worth the wait. Don't give up.

***Note: This book is self-published and self-edited. My apologies for any grammatical errors and using the occasional infertility-induced swear word. Please blame the side effects of my fertility medications.

About this Book

Infertility is a series of moments. The moment you start trying for your baby. The moment of anticipation before you see the results of a pregnancy test. The moment you meet with a fertility doctor for the first time. The moment you try IUI or IVF. The moment you think you're pregnant or know that you're not. There are moments of uncertainty, desperation and confusion. Moments of disappointment, anger and envy. Moments of intense happiness; hopefulness and joy; optimism; elation and strength.

In your journey towards parenthood, you probably wouldn't include laughter and humor as part of these moments. Infertility, itself, is not funny. It is difficult and heartbreaking and painful. But through life's uncertainty, you can still find humor through challenges. I dare you to laugh at infertility. I dare you to find humor in all the crazy things you do to get pregnant. I dare you to step out of the darkness and learn to smile again.

Nope. Trying to make a baby is not funny at all. There is nothing funny about putting three pillows under your ass and keeping your legs elevated after baby-making sex. There is definitely nothing hilarious about holding your husband's semen analysis cup under your bra so you could keep it warm for your IUI. And there is nothing funny about accidentally saying the word 'ovulation' during a staff meeting or in front of your boss.

I started writing my blog, '999 Reasons to Laugh at Infertility,' when I realized that I had forgotten how to laugh during my long battle with infertility. Five years ago, on one deliciously warm and sexy evening, my husband turned to me and said, *"honey, let's make a baby tonight."* We had just celebrated our two year wedding anniversary and with my birthday quickly approaching, my biological clock reminded me that I wasn't getting any younger. We were in our late twenties and it felt like the right time to start trying. At the time, I had no idea when my peak ovulation cycle was; I didn't know what TTC meant and I didn't even know that I had a basal temperature. I had no idea what infertility was. That fateful evening, we tossed out the condoms, giggled hysterically and started trying to make our baby. Twenty eight days later I got my period. A monthly visitor that would show up uninvited for the next five years.

After a couple months of trying, I wasn't discouraged. After all, my friends had told me that it took them several months to get pregnant. In my head, I had a few more months of trying before it was my turn. But many months later, my bathroom had turned into a fertility laboratory filled with ovulation sticks, a basal thermometer, and a garbage can filled with negative pregnancy tests. It seemed like all my friends had gotten pregnant and I was the only one left behind. Every pregnancy announcement transformed me into a jealous person and I secretly hated attending baby showers and reading Facebook status updates about pregnancy.

My husband and I quickly found ourselves in a new world dominated by the fertility clinic. A strange new place filled with early morning blood and ultrasound appointments; awkward conversations about my husband's (lack of) semen; and costly fertility bills. *"Doctor, you want to stick that transvaginal wand WHERE?"* Suddenly, my world was a place of negative moments, depression and hopelessness.

Then one day, I had enough. I found strength. Ironically, I found my hope while sitting on the toilet seat, feeling depressed. *What am I doing?* I thought to myself. *Who have I become?* I was tired of crying. Tired of feeling depressed and angry. Tired of feeling jealous and sorry for myself. I knew I needed to change my attitude and find happiness again. In that moment, I decided to stop crying. I had put my life on hold for infertility for far too long, and I refused to pause my life any longer. I had wasted so many months crying that I was missing out on living. I refused to let infertility weigh me down, and I decided that laughing was more fun than feeling depressed about my situation. I started my blog and challenged myself to think of 999 reasons to laugh at infertility.

And somehow, amidst all the baby showers, fertility drugs, baby announcements and negative pregnancy tests, I began to smile again. I was determined to be a mother and I refused to give up hope of becoming a parent. Two IUIs and four IVF cycles later, I kicked some infertility ass! I got pregnant through IVF and became a mommy to a beautiful baby boy.

You have choices in life. You can either hide in the shadows or learn to dance in the rain. You can either spend your time thinking about everything you don't have or enjoy everything you do. Everyone goes through difficult life challenges but you have the power to change your attitude. You are not alone. Life does not stop for infertility. Laugh, smile and be determined, and remember that, "Everything will be okay in the end. If it's not okay, it's not the end."

xoxo,
Semi-Infertile Naomi
Twitter @InfertileNaomi

Fertility Acronym Decoder

Welcome to the confusing world of fertility acronyms where BFN no longer stands for Big Fabulous Nachos and IVF doesn't mean I'm Very Fertile.

AF ~ Aunt Flow

AI ~ Artificial Insemination

AID ~ Artificial Insemination from Donor

BD ~ Baby Dance

BBT ~ Basal Body Temperature

BCP ~ Birth Control Pills

Beta, HCG ~ Pregnancy blood test

BG ~ Blood Glucose

BW ~ Blood work

BFN ~ Big Fat Negative

BFP ~ Big Fat Positive

CD ~ Cycle Day

CF ~ Cervical Fluid

CM ~ Cervical Mucus

CNM ~ Certified Nurse Midwife

COH ~ Controlled Ovarian Hyper stimulation

CP ~ Cervical Position

DH ~ Darling Husband

DD ~ Darling Daughter

DS ~ Darling Son

D&C ~ Dilation and Curettage

D&E ~ Dilation and Evacuation

DE ~ Donor Eggs

DI ~ Donor Insemination

DPO ~ Days Past Ovulation

EDD ~ Estimated Due Date

ENDO ~ Endometriosis

EPT ~ Early Pregnancy Test

ERT ~ Estrogen Replacement Therapy

FP ~ Follicular Phase

FHR ~ Follicle Stimulating Hormone

FMU ~ First Morning Urine

FM ~ Fertility Monitor

GP ~ General Practitioner

HCG ~ Human Chronic Gonadotropin

HCP ~ Health Care Practitioner

HPT ~ Home Pregnancy Test

HRT ~ Hormone Replacement Therapy

HSC ~ Hysteroscopy

HSG ~ Hysterosalpingogram

IF ~ Infertility

IVF ~ In Vitro Fertilization

IUI ~ Inter Uterine Insemination

LAP ~ Laparoscopy

LH ~ Luteinzing Hormone

LMP ~ Last Menstrual Period

LP ~ Luteal Phase

2WW ~ 2 Week Wait

LSP ~ Low Sperm Count

MC ~ Miscarriage

MF ~ Male Factor

NP ~ Nurse Practitioner

OV ~ Ovulation

OC ~ Oral Contraceptives

OHSS ~ Ovarian Hyperstimulation Syndrome

OPK ~ Ovulation Predictor Kit

P4 ~ Progesterone

PCO ~ Polycystic Ovaries

PCOS ~ Polycystic Ovarian Syndrome

PCP ~ Primary Care Physician

PG ~ Pregnant

PI ~ Primary Infertility

PID ~ Pelvic Inflammatory Disease

PMS ~ Premenstrual Syndrome

RE ~ Reproductive Endocrinologist

RI ~ Reproductive Immunologist

SA ~ Semen Analysis

SI ~ Secondary Infertility

TTC ~ Trying to conceive

TL ~ Tubal Ligation

TR ~ Tubal Reversal

UR ~ Urologist

US ~ Ultrasound

V ~ Vasectomy

VR ~ Vasectomy Reversal

Don't Forget These Other Uncommon (But More Fun) Fertility Acronyms

IHFPU ~ I hate Facebook pregnancy updates.

WTFAINPY ~ Why the fertile am I not pregnant yet?

ITOPWIP ~ I'm the only person who isn't pregnant!

MFAAPAAMEAITF ~ My friends are all pregnant and all my embryos are in the freezer.

ICEGPWTPTSRITE ~ I can't even get pregnant when they put the sperm right into the egg!

WIOB ~ Where is our baby?

IDWTHYPN ~ I don't want to hear your pregnancy news.

CMIMFTOM ~ Cervical mucus is my favorite type of mucus!

WRAIDH ~ We relaxed and it didn't happen.

PTATD ~ Pregnancy tests are the devil.

IGHOFA ~ I get high on folic acid.

MHHADBTDMOC ~ My husband has a damn business trip during my ovulation cycle!

ILAMVDMTILAMH ~ I look at my vaginal discharge more than I look at my husband.

IWSMFCIIHT ~ I will stalk my fertility clinic if I have to!

MLSGPBMAIJ ~ My little sister got pregnant before me and I'm jealous.

IWTKYBBIKTTIMH ~ I want to keep your baby but I keep that thought in my head.

WSHH ~ We still have hope.

WWNGU ~ We will never give up!

"Don't ask a woman if she is pregnant unless her water breaks on your flip-flops, a baby arm dangles out of her vagina and she asks you to cut the cord and then and only then may you ask if she's having a baby. Otherwise, shut up." ~Actress Nia Vardalos

Reason to Laugh at Infertility #1
You Google Words Like 'Ovulation' and 'Am I Pregnant?'

The internet is both a terrible and wonderful tool for finding information about infertility. There is a lot of helpful information but also many scam websites that promise miracle infertility cures. But like many other people struggling with infertility, you spend your time behind the monitor asking Doctor Google about your possible pregnancy symptoms. You spend many hours googling questions like, 'I have a fever during my two week wait. Is that a pregnancy symptom?' and 'I just peed four times, does that mean I'm pregnant?' and 'will forcing my husband to eat walnuts improve his low sperm count?'

If you find yourself googling strange fertility questions on the internet, you are not alone. We all do it. Chances are, you have probably googled one or all of the following searches in the privacy of your own house (or even at your workplace):

- Doctor Google, does IVF drugs make me constipated?
- Doctor Google, will my hysterosalpingogram be any fun?
- Does crying excessively after failing an IVF burn calories?
- I just deleted all my pregnant Facebook friends. Is that wrong?
- Why is my younger sister pregnant before me?
- If I re-pee on a pregnancy test, will that make it positive?
- My right breast feels more swollen then my left, am I pregnant?
- How do I get pregnant like the Octomom?

Be warned. Google might respond and say, "stop googling your possible pregnancy symptoms, you crazy infertile! I have no idea if you're pregnant or not!"

#2 You Examine the Toilet Paper

A Toilet Paper Examiner, Noun
Definition: The act of (excessively) examining the toilet paper every time you go to the bathroom for signs of ovulation or your period.

Infertility has turned you into a 'Toilet Paper Examiner.' Before you were trying to conceive, you use to go to the bathroom, and toss away the toilet paper without even a second glance. Now, you inspect every corner of that toilet paper, searching for signs of your period and/or cervical mucus. You examine the toilet paper while asking yourself questions like, 'is this really my period or is this just spotting?' Unfortunately, if you don't lock the bathroom door, your husband might walk into the room as you are wiping and inspecting. Don't bother explaining. He won't really understand. On one occasion, you thought you saw blood on the toilet paper a week before your period was expected to arrive. You got extremely excited, believing that it might be implantation bleeding and then realized that it was, sadly, just blood from shaving your legs. It's official, infertility has made you weird. Fertility Tip: Purchase toilet paper in bulk.

#3 You Trick Your Basal Thermometer

You do it every morning. You get out of bed, sit on the toilet seat and take your basal temperature. You stick that pink thermometer into your mouth with a silent prayer that your temperature will remain elevated. You feel a sense of elation when you see your temperature spike; and when it begins to drop, so does your heart. That's when you do whatever it takes to trick the thermometer! You might try to take your temperature at different times of the day when you know your temp. will be elevated. You take it after a hot bath, after a workout, stepping out of the shower or after drinking a cup of hot tea. Congratulations! Your temperature is now elevated! You may even decide to remove the thermometer from your mouth when you notice things aren't going your way. The thermometer seems to be increasing too slowly which means your temperature is dropping. Yikes! Fertility Tip: Remove the thermometer right away and keep your sanity!

#4 You Analyze Your Breasts for Early Pregnancy Symptoms

It is one week before your expected period and you truly believe that your breasts will tell you the answer. Am I pregnant? You give your breasts a better examination than a doctor giving a mammogram. First, you check yourself out in the mirror to examine those boobies in all their glory. Your right breast seems to be heavier than your left breast. Your breasts feel more tender and sore than usual. You wonder if this is an early pregnancy symptom. Yes, your right side is definitely more tender. You quickly google, 'tender breasts one week before period.' You find a slew of google answers and a couple of them tell you that you might be pregnant!

You may even ask your husband if your breasts look larger. He takes a look but doesn't give you the answer you want to hear. *"Sorry honey, your boobs look the same to me."* Wrong answer, husband. Wrong answer.

And don't forget about those nipples. You have never examined your nipples so much in your life. *Are my nipples looking a little too brown or more pink? I swear that my nipple looks different today...I think.* You also google, 'darker colored nipples, early pregnancy symptom?' The Google Doctor tells you again you might be pregnant. You love this doctor! But then you get your period, and your breasts stop hurting immediately. Stupid Google Doctors.

#5 You Have Pregnancy Books on Your Nightstand

If you are trying to conceive, you probably have at least two pregnancy and/or fertility books by your bedside. These books are either (a) hidden in a drawer (underneath the unused box of expired condoms), or (b) scattered under your bed away from sight. You don't really want guests stumbling into your bedroom and finding these books one day. You love reading pregnancy books but you ALWAYS turn to the 'trying to conceive' and 'infertility' chapters first. You have even asked your husband to read the section about male factor infertility (he skimmed it briefly).

You have picked up these books at your local bookstore or at the library, always a little embarrassed to purchase them from the cashier. You don't have anything to feel ashamed about but you still would rather not discuss it in public. Sometimes you just browse the bookstore for hours, flipping through books without actually buying it. You look around the bookstore cautiously to make sure you don't run into anyone before picking up a book.

If you do run into someone, this is what might happen:

Friend: *"(Insert your name here) Is that you?"*

You: (Quickly hide ovulation book) *"Oh hi. What are you doing here?"*

Friend: *"I'm looking for a pregnancy book. I just found out I'm pregnant!"*

You: (monotone) *"Congratulations. Neat-o news."*

Friend: (looks down at your belly) *"Are you pregnant too?"*

You: *"I just remembered, I have to go."* (Unsure of what to say, you throw your ovulation and cervical mucus book on the floor and run to the bathroom where you cry for at least thirty minutes. Your entire day is ruined).

"Life isn't about trying to weather the storm. It's about learning to dance in the rain." ~Vivian Greene

#6 Vacation Sex Didn't Work

Everyone advises you to 'just relax and it will happen.' Oh sure. You really believe that. How could you possibly relax? You're not getting any younger here and your eggs are aging a little more each day. You have avoided that much needed vacation due to fertility appointments and cycle monitoring for months but now it's time to try baby-making vacation sex! Your friends have told you endless stories about how they knew someone (who knew someone else) who had been trying for years and got pregnant after a trip to Mexico. Apparently, your friend's cousin's hairdresser had vacation sex and came home pregnant with twins! Maybe that will happen to you!

You leave for your vacation feeling relaxed and (somewhat) confident you will come home pregnant. You and your husband have a great trip with tons of baby-making sex. All fertility rules are thrown out the window – you can have sex multiple times a day and you hope your husband's sperm count will still remain plentiful. So when Aunt Flow arrives that following month, you are somewhat surprised. You start to think of excuses why you didn't get knocked up. It must have been that two hour time change that made a difference to your internal clock or perhaps your body didn't adjust well to all that new food. That's what it was, for sure. Well, at least you had a great trip and spent money on something other than fertility treatments.

#7 You are Envious of Morning Sickness

You know you're obsessed with pregnancy when even morning sickness sounds good to you. But does it really? Any pregnant woman would tell you otherwise. Excessive vomiting, non-stop diarrhea, nausea, laying on the bathroom floor begging for saltine crackers. That sounds absolutely fantastic! To anyone struggling with infertility, the mere thought of any pregnancy symptom makes you feel happy, even morning sickness. Suddenly one morning, you too feel nauseated and are (somewhat) excited thinking you might be pregnant. You get sick from last night's Chinese food and you happily rush to take your basal temperature. You couldn't be more overjoyed! But then your period arrives shortly afterwards, and you feel confused. Was it morning sickness or maybe that chicken was a bit undercook? It's okay to be envious of morning sickness. One day, you hope to experience it too (or maybe just light nausea instead). You've been through enough already.

#8 You Did a Headstand After Baby-Making Sex

You could have been a gymnast or at least a member of Cirque du Soleil. You really missed your calling. Your doctor recommended putting a pillow under your behind and elevating your legs for thirty minutes after baby-making sex. No urinating either, ladies (a mistake you made several times, early on!).

Following baby-making sex, you have tried:

- A full headstand.
- A partial headstand where you placed your hands on your lower back and lifted your legs straight above your head.
- Lifting your pelvis.
- Putting TWO or THREE pillows under your behind (the recommended one pillow is not working out for you).
- Laying on the bedroom floor and placing your legs on the wall.
- Any other yoga pose.

Your husband continues to be impressed during each of your Cirque du Soleil performances. If anyone is interested in buying tickets, your next morning performance is twelve days after your next period.

#9 Your Mom Clips Out Newspaper Articles About Infertility

Thanks mother. I just LOVED the article you gave me about how to increase my fertility. Every time you go to your parent's house, there seems to be a fertility-related article clipped out just for you. Your mom has made it her mission to clip out any and every newspaper article about infertility on your behalf. Mommy typically pulls you aside and whispers in your ear, *"honey, there is a newspaper article for you upstairs."* Sometimes she'll send you an email too – *"Remind me to give you a newspaper article when you come over tomorrow."*
Thank a lot mother.

But chances are, if she saw the article, you did too. You are secretly (or not so secretly) obsessed with those articles as well. *"Honey, have you ever charted your temperature using something called a basal thermometer?"* your mom will innocently inquire. Yes mother. I have been recording my temperature for two years now but thanks. *"Honey, do you know when you're ovulating?"* Yes mother. Please stop asking me this. *"Honey, have you ever asked your doctor about PCOS?"* Yes mother. But I do not have PCOS. You gotta love mothers. One day, when you become a mom, you will probably do the same thing to your kid. And you cannot wait!

#10 You Touched Your Own Cervix

Did you know that you can actually touch your own cervix to predict ovulation? If you are struggling with infertility, you have probably already tried this. When you first met your husband, you were shy about doing number two in front of him. Now, you go into your bathroom and try to touch your cervix whether he is home or not. You have no shame left. *"Sweetheart! Someone's on the telephone for you,"* your husband shouts while you're in the bathroom. What can you say? *"I'll call them back. I only have one hand available right now!"*

A friend recommended you read a fertility book claiming that it was 'life changing.' Your friend, who got pregnant within four months, said that it helped her. You read it anyways, hoping the book would help you conceive. It didn't. But the author did provide a detailed account about how to properly touch your cervix:

As you approach ovulation, your cervix will become soft to the touch. It begins by feeling firm like the tip of your nose and when you're ovulating, your cervix will feel soft like your lips. Go ahead, put the book down and touch it!.

Wow. That sounds like so much fun! Fertility Tip: Touching your cervix in your workplace toilet is not recommended.

"Nature has got it all wrong: When you are younger, it should be harder to get pregnant, and as you get older it should be easier. When you are so ready, you can't do it to save your life. And when you are 21, you are so not ready, but you are ripe as could be. The eggs should become more developed the older you get, not die slowly from the day you're born. That's one thing God got wrong." ~Actress Halle Berry

#11 Your Friend Announced Her Pregnancy at a Restaurant

Which is better? Learning a friend is pregnant before or after you eat? You meet your gal pal for lunch and she excitedly blurts out the news that she is eating for two. Inside, a deep, familiar sadness pounds in your chest. Your eyes quietly water behind your lids. Your inner voice says, *'I started trying months ago. How did she get pregnant so quickly. Why isn't it me?'* But your outer, rational voice says, *"oh my gosh. I am so happy for you. You look great. You're not even showing yet."*

Now it's time to look at the menu. She is famished but you are a different story. You now have either lost your appetite completely or you are trying to find the most unhealthy item on the menu. The caffeine vodka chocolate cake looks tasty. Most likely, your appetite is ruined and you feel terrible for secretly feeling so selfish. You were starving a minute ago and now you don't know if you can even stomach bread and water.

If only she had waited until after the meal to tell you the news. You probably would have felt sick to your stomach anyways. Now, you have to make small chat, eat your meal and then have your complete breakdown in the car ride home. Fertility Tip: When the restaurant bill arrives, let her treat.

#12 Your Dentist Has Becomes the Fertility Expert

You go to many different physicians; the eye doctor, the dentist, the allergist and you wait for that one question the doctor always asks: *"Are you taking any medications?"* You dread this question because it always results in the same answer. You are taking prenatal vitamins, fertility drugs and no doctor, I AM NOT PREGNANT. You always have to further explain that you have been trying for a long time and it hasn't happened yet. Your doctor will then take it upon himself to offer you unwanted fertility advice.

"Just relax and it will just happen," doctor allergist will advise. Thanks a lot Mr. Allergist but just concentrate on my ragweed sensitivity. It gets even more difficult as time goes on and you see the same doctor on a regular basis. You are forced to have the same conversation again and then listen to the same advise. *"You're STILL trying for a baby?"* doctor teeth will ask. *"Have you tired to relax?"* No offense doctor, you are no fertility specialist. Please just remove my cavity in silence.

#13 Your Baby Nursery is Now Your Office

When you first moved into your new house, you imagined having a nursery for your future child. You know which room it is. It's the middle room just beside your bedroom so you could check on your baby frequently. You would walk past this room several times a day, and picture a crib and a rocking chair. You would stand in the doorway and imagine yourself rocking your baby to sleep and seeing that room filled with little clothes and toys. You even painted the room a baby friendly color (without mentioning this intent to your husband). But now, this room has become your office.

Instead of plush animals and baby dresses, this room now has a desk, an old chair, a computer and a scatter of pens and papers. The image of a sweet crib has been replaced by a mountain of paperwork and you now have photos of other people's children on your desk.Perhaps one day this will be your baby's room but for now, it's the room where you spend hours looking at infertility websites and nursing back a martini.

#14 You Pretend Your Friend's Baby is Your Own

Is it wrong to pretend that a friend's baby is your own? You are at the shopping mall and your friend asks you to look after her baby while she runs to the toilet. Dangerous.Very dangerous. Never leave your child alone with a crazy infertile. You happily agree to look after the kid but in the back of your mind, you pretend that it's your child. You might even hope to run into someone you know. You would just wave from a distance and happily push the stroller like all the other fake mothers do.

Another time, you spend the afternoon holding your friend's baby. You glance at your husband and imagine that this is your child. You can pretty much guarantee that your husband is not thinking the same thing. Even a (crazy) infertile knows that stealing a baby is wrong but pretending that your friend's child is your own baby is completely healthy. Right? Mommy friends beware.

#15 Surviving the Dreaded Baby Shower Party

That adorable, pink invitation arrives in the mail and your heart drops. You know exactly what it is:

THE DREADED BABY SHOWER INVITATION.

Here are some helpful tips for surviving the baby shower party:

- Arrive in tears. You are going to spend most of the baby shower crying in the bathroom anyways so why not make it a public event?

- Start telling other guests about your struggles with infertility and don't forget to be very detailed about ovulation and cervical mucus.

- Bring a cake that says: Congratulations! It took you less than a year to conceive!

- Leave a negative pregnancy test and a package of birth control pills in her bathroom.

- Introduce inappropriate party games including, 'Guess the baby daddy' and 'Pin the tail on the cervix.'

- Yawn loudly during present opening and ask if you can take a nap in her bed.

- Put a sign on her front door that reads, Baby shower canceled due to marital break-up.

"Hope is a renewable option: If you run out of it at the end of the day, you get to start over in the morning." ~Barbara Kingsolver

#16 Everyone on Facebook is Pregnant

In the pre-Facebook days, infertile women were tortured from seeing pregnant women on the street. Now, you get to be tortured through technology as well. Out of your six hundred 'friends' on Facebook, at least half are pregnant or just given birth. It begins with the three month belly pictures where friends comment their congratulations, and preggy's profile turns into an ultrasound photo. Each month, new pictures surface of the belly, and you wish you didn't turn on your computer.

Pregnancy status updates begin! *"Yuck. I feel so sick today!"* and *"my feet are so swollen. It's awful."* You refuse to comment on their updates but you can't help and look at the photos. There's the twelve week ultrasound photo! There's the six month belly shot! Neat-o! Thankfully, no one can see your jealousy through the computer screen.

And eventually, when your friend gives birth, don't expect a personal phone call. She will just update her Facebook page. *"We're now three and it's a HE! Welcome Baby Bart to the world!"* Watch for new photos of the baby to appear daily.

Monday's photo: Bart's first poopie diaper
Tuesday: Bart's first burpie
Wednesday: Bart picks his nose
Thursday: Bart gets a bum rash
Friday: Bart's first trip at the zoo
Then, another Facebook friend announces a pregnancy and the cycle starts again. Thank goodness for the friend delete button! Don't be afraid to use it.

Often.

#17 IVF: The Cookbook

From the bestselling IVF Cookbook: A Scrambled Egg Recipe
Prep/Conception Time: 1-10 years.
Cost: $10,000. Materials not included.

INGREDIENTS
- 8-12 ripe follicles
- 8-12 hard boiled eggs
- 50 million sperms (washed)
- 5-10 fertility drugs and vitamins
- 2-5 nurses/fertility interns
- 1 tiny test tube (sterilized)

DIRECTIONS
- Crack open your legs and enjoy an internal massage for 30 minutes, daily.
- Combine fertility medications until properly digested.
- Draw blood at the clinic, daily.
- Spread legs, finely.
- Remove eggs. Do not chop.
- Rub male parts until explosive results. Wash contents immediately.
- Mix eggs with white content in a small dish. Keep warm.
- Drizzle filling into small opening.
- When ready to serve, insert, then let cool for 30 minutes. Insert panty liner.
- Garnish as necessary. Serve fresh or frozen.

Makes: 1- Octuplet Servings.

Recipe Reviews - 3 stars ***
Sarah said: *I tried this costly dish at least 6 times this year!*
Becky said: *I failed at it. I never want to make this again!*
Lauren said: *My husband felt that he could have made more.*
Katie said: *I wouldn't recommend it to any of my friends. I felt ill after.*
Samantha said: *My third attempt resulted in 8 more mouths to feed.*

#18 Your Secret Infertile Inner Thoughts

Positive affirmations. You have read the book, The Secret, and know that if you really believe something will happen, it will. Oprah Winfrey says so. People have told you that if you believe you will get pregnant, then it will happen. So why hasn't it yet? In the inner workings of your infertile mind, you try to repeat positive pregnancy affirmations in hopes that your womb will somehow hear your message.

I will get pregnant. I will be a mother. I will have a baby this year. I will carry a child to term. I will keep saying these positive pregnancy affirmations so my partner's sperm will somehow get the message. You hear me, low motility sperm count!

After an IUI, it may look like you are laying on your back with your eyes shut but you are actually meditating. If only the nurse knew what you were really thinking. *His sperm is strong and plentiful. My uterus is a happy and inviting place. I will ovulate and reproduce.* After baby-making sex, your partner is happily sleeping while you lay on your back in an elevated position for the next thirty minutes. Meditation begins.

My partner's sperm has only one tail and head. My cervical mucus is a warm and sperm-healthy environment. My fallopian tubes are open and clear.

Good thing no one can hear what you're thinking! Yikes!

#19 People Tell You to 'Just Adopt'

Don't say the 'A' word in front of you. You are not ready to hear it. There are some people who choose adoption as their first choice and others based on circumstance. Then, there are others (maybe like yourself) who can't yet bring themselves to even think about adoption. You believe that adoption is a wonderful thing but not sure if it's right for you. You may believe that discussing adoption is like giving up the idea of ever becoming pregnant. You may feel open to adoption but can't explore it just yet. Now, the mere reference to, 'why don't you just adopt?' gets your blood boiling.

"Our neighbor just adopted and then they got pregnant," your friend says. Good for your neighbors. *"Have you ever considered adoption? Angelina and Brad did it,"* your ditzy cousin says. You instantly hate her. You are willing to adopt a pet, adapt to a new job, adept to a new skill but adoption? You are still not there yet. Right now, you are just going to adopt this cup of delicious caffeinated coffee.

#20 The Security Guard Found an Ovulation Stick in Your Purse

The last thing you need is someone searching though your purse, filled with medication and other fertility goodies. But it's inevitable. You go to a concert, you go through airport security and someone has to search your hand bag. They may be searching for weapons but what they'll find is something very very different.

BEEP! BEEP! BEEP! The sensors go off and the security guard needs to search your bag. *"Lady, what the HECK is this?"*

Oh, Mr. Security Guard, it's only a package of ovulation predictor kits, a pregnancy test, a container of fertility pills, a basal thermometer, a temperature chart, dixie pee cups, an RE business card, a donor egg, a package of washed sperm, raspberry leaf tea, a fertility DVD, a saliva ovulation detector, and one or two (just in case) tampons. What seems to be the problem?

Fertility Tip: When going through security, it's probably a good idea to remove your fertility needle and your ovulation chart from your purse.

"Don't cry over spilt milk (unless you're crying because you don't have breast milk, then it's okay to cry.)" ~Infertile Naomi, a woman who relaxed and it didn't happen

#21 You Peed After Baby-Making Sex

At the beginning, you had no idea that it wasn't recommended to pee following sex. There were many times when you happily rushed off to the toilet after an adventurous baby-making experience. Your future children poured out of you and quietly drowned into the toilet bowl. Bad, bad mother. Later, when you started waiting the recommended thirty minutes before going to the bathroom, you thought back to all your sweet potential children that met their early death by toilet water.

You shudder when you think of the time your potential child dripped down your leg or met their death in a puddle in your panties. The time you let out a loud cough, and a gush of sperm stained your bed or perhaps, the time you wiped the remaining liquid on a piece of toilet paper. Watching your future sperm babies helplessly drown in a toilet bowl is terribly sad. A good (and crazy) mother would have saved them and stuck them back inside.

#22 You Tested Early Because You Wanted to Surprise Your Husband

As William Shakespeare once (sort of) said, *'To test or not to test, that is the question.'* You have survived the dreaded two week wait and you still have a couple more days until it's okay to take a pregnancy test. You really want to test early. Could it really hurt to test a couple of days early? Let me make the answer easier for you: DON'T TEST EARLY!

A lot of thoughts go through your infertile mind:

- If I test today and it's positive, I can surprise my husband on his birthday
- I had a really hard day and this is the only thing that will make me happy.
- Imagine if I tested positive and I can surprise my husband on our anniversary!

All those thoughts are really great but only if the test comes back positive. If it comes back negative (like it typically does), your hubby's birthday is now ruined; and you can now enjoy a mental breakdown instead of dinner and a movie on your anniversary. Fertility Tip: Whatever you do, don't test early. Just hold onto hope for one more day.

#23 You Mark Your Ovulation Dates on Your Calendar

Check your calendar. Lunch with Mindy on Tuesday, book club on Friday, ovulate on Sunday. If someone looked at your calendar right now, they would know when you're due to ovulate. Actually, if someone looked back at your calendar for the last six months, they would know all your recent menstrual cycles and ovulation dates.

The fertility doctor wants to know when your last period was. Well, that's easy! Just look it up on your calendar! Planning a business trip? Just schedule it around those ovulation dates. A shared calendar is also great so your husband/partner will always know when he will 'get some' or when you are scheduled to burst into tears.

No, I can't get together next Tuesday, Sally. I am supposed to spend that entire day crying and feeling miserable. How about lunch on Friday instead? Fertility Tip: Charting your ovulation and period dates on a shared work calendar is not recommended.

#24 How to Cheat on an IUI

Congratulations! You failed your first IUI or IVF treatment! Hurts pretty bad, doesn't it? You are now onto your second (or seventh) treatment and you will go into this cycle a little less optimistic, believing that it probably won't work, if it didn't work the first time. Do you really think you can cheat on your next IUI/IVF and outsmart your body?

If you are a true infertile, some of these ideas might have crossed your mind.

1. Get your husband/partner to drink extra coffee before doing his business. You think that if he's more alert, then his little guys will be too.

2. Eat an entire pineapple during your two week wait because you read somewhere that it strengthens your uterine lining.

3. Refuse to exercise during your two week wait although your doctor recommends the opposite.

4. Put at least twenty pillows under your behind following the procedure.

5. Before the procedure, have a chat with his sperm.

6. Slip the fertility nurse $50.00 to give you a positive.

7. Bring in some cheat sheets to your procedure.

8. Take the catheter home with you and insert any leftovers yourself.

9. Refuse to cough or fart for the next twenty-four hours in fear your baby will squirt out.

10. Pretend not to think about pregnancy during your two week wait.

Yes, future children. Cheating is a good thing.

#25 The 'Just Relax and It Will Happen' Response

Infertility is the invisible ailment. No one talks about it and no one knows how to respond to it. You often get the 'just relax and it will happen' useless response, the 'I feel so bad for you' pity look or the 'I don't know what to say and I'm uncomfortable' reaction. These people typically wait for you to bring up the subject although you know they are dying to say something. You can see it in their eyes. Should I ask her about her broken uterus? Should I wait for her to say something first?

And when you do bring up the subject, you can see pity in their eyes. They automatically offer you fertility advice or tell you a success story of someone they know who got pregnant. *"So and so tried this product and she got pregnant." "I heard this fertility book* (insert random book title) *was really good. You should read it."* They try to be helpful but you wish they were better listeners than talkers.

And of course, you also know the infertility gossiper who tells you to 'just relax and it will happen' and you will definitely 'be the next one to get pregnant.' She treats your news like a good piece of gossip, asking questions and giving useless advice. Well guess what? We relaxed and it didn't happen! But don't feel sorry for us! We are obviously incredibly happy and stable women, who are clearly not depressed, upset or irrational about our situation at all. Clearly.

#26 You Haven't Ovulated Since the 1990s

It is the early 1990s. The real 90210 is on television, Madonna tops the charts, you are crushing on Doogie Howser M.D., the world is fearful about Y2K and you have only ovulated once in the past five years. While other women get their periods on a regular twenty-eight day cycle, you have only seen Aunt Flow a few times a year. You enjoy her arrival because that means you actually have a chance this month. In your situation, you probably need medical assistance to actually bring on ovulation and sometimes it works but more often, it doesn't.

You feel guilty that your body doesn't work properly and blame yourself for not getting pregnant. Ovulation predictor kits are your best friend, (if you could friend them on Facebook, you would). When your fertility doctor tells you it's time to ovulate, you rush home and get the job done! When that doesn't work, you say goodbye to Ms. Ovulation again and hope to see her soon. If only that hunky Doogie Howser, M.D. was a fertility specialist. You'd let him check out your cervix anytime.

"If you can't find hope, look in a new direction." ~unknown

#27 You Pre-Failed Your IUI

Only an infertile could pre-fail an IUI or IVF cycle before it even happened. Your procedure is scheduled for next Thursday but you already 'know' that it didn't work. You just know that his sperm count will be low, the medications won't work, that your cycle will be canceled. In your mind, it's like you predict disappointment because it will ease your pain later on. News flash! A negative pregnancy test still hurts like a bitch!

You were hopeful during your first IUI or IVF, but once you got to number two or three or ten, optimism flew out the window. Why bother eating healthy? Why continue to take prenatal pills? Have a cup of extra strong caffeinated coffee! You already know the outcome anyways.

You: *"Honey, sorry to tell you but we failed our IUI. I just know I'm not pregnant this month"*
Husband: *"But our IUI is not until next week."*

It takes a special person to pre-fail a fertility procedure before it has even occurred.

#28 Your Fertility Drugs are in the Refrigerator

Move over meatloaf and leftover casserole. Make room for your fertility medication! Hungry? Should you have a piece of fruit, some cheese or a gulp of delicious Puregon? During dinner parties, you hope your guests will not rummage through your fridge because that isn't a bottle of sparkling water! That's your special fertility drink! What should you have for breakfast today? Maybe some scrambled eggs with a side of fertility needle?

Your refrigerator has become your instant infertility reminder. You open up that fridge in the morning and see your meds before grabbing that container of milk. Your fridge automatically screams at you: NOT PREGNANT! NOT PREGNANT! It is the only appliance in your house that can make you feel as depressed as the arrival of Auntie Flow. Shut up fridge! Now, if your toaster oven or microwave starts reminding you of infertility, you might want to check with a fertility (or mental health) specialist.

#29 The Screw You Fertility Diet

You've tried a fertility-friendly diet. When you first started trying, you gave up caffeine, stopped drinking diet sodas, and stocked up on those recommended dark, leafy greens. How did that work out for you? Not so well? It seems that other women can have a completely unhealthy diet and get pregnant easily, or worse get pregnant just 'by accident.' It's just not fair. Then, as time goes on, your 'fertility-friendly' diet turned into the 'who cares I'm not getting pregnant anyways' diet.

Hello caffeinated coffee! Good morning chocolate! Ola artificial sweeteners! No complete servings of fruits and vegetables for you! Maybe you'll have two glasses of wine with dinner. And watch out during Aunt Flow days! No Folic Acid for you! You know what? You are trying to do the best you can. You adapted the fertility-friendly diet and it didn't work. Fertility Tip: That teenage girl didn't get pregnant because she ate her dark leafy greens for dinner. Eat healthy, take your Folic Acid, have the occasional yummy treat and enjoy your life. You deserve it.

#30 You Stare at Baby Strollers

You may have a dislike for pregnant bellies but you sure do love those babies! Mom alert ahead....She's pushing a stroller....She walks by you....(wait for it).... It's time for you to look at that baby....You turn around to get a glimpse of the baby....You smile and think how cute that baby is....Then you feel sad...Where is your baby? Two moms ahead...Pushing newborn strollers....You're dying to look in....They pass by you....Turn your head to look....So cute. Fresh out the womb....You wish one of those babies were yours.

A pregnant woman walks by and you're certain she can feel the envy in your eyes and the bitter breeze of your stare but a baby goes by and you can't help but smile. Tears fill your eyes with love. Maybe next time you see a stroller coming, you should tell that woman she has a beautiful baby and she was so lucky that she was able to conceive. Then, ask her politely, if you could just have her baby. Maybe she'll give it to you (or runaway in fear). Fertility Tip: Don't let an infertile near your stroller. She will want to take the baby home with her and she won't bring it back.

#31 The Pity Invitation From Your Mommy Friends

The childless couple gets all the pity invitations. *"It's little Jenny's first birthday party on Saturday but I'll understand if you don't want to come."* When you do attend the birthday parties, you and your partner sit at the singles table, making awkward small chat with her never-been-married Aunt Ruth and the one other potentially infertile couple. Seeing all those babies makes you further depressed and you leave the party, feeling like you're never going to get pregnant. Happy f---ing first birthday, little Jenny. Sigh.

You find that you either get the pity invitation or you don't get invited to the party at all. The infertile couple doesn't get invited to the Halloween party, the Christmas party or the mommy get together held every Thursday. You watch from the bleachers as all your mommy friends take their kids to the circus, kiddie concerts and the zoo. You aren't invited but you get the added bonus of hearing about it later through Facebook photos in an album called, 'Here are all the parties you weren't invited to.'

It's so thoughtful that you were invited to all the pre-baby parties including the baby shower and the 'I'm pregnant and you're not' dinner parties. Maybe you can return the favor and invite your fertile friends to your latest IUI party, 'My follicles are growing in a test tube' celebration or 'I just paid $10,000 for a failed cycle' blowout. Kids are not welcome. In leu of gifts, please give alcohol.

#32 You Started Wearing Maxi Pads Again

Remember the day your fourteen year old self first discovered tampons? You realized that you no longer had to wear those uncomfortable fitting pads and discovered that tampons were easy and clean and great. Twenty years later, infertility re-introduces the sanitary napkin! Somewhere during your infertility struggles, you may decide to switch back to pads, even for one month. It's unclear if tampons actually affect fertility but an infertile will try anything even if it means sitting in a wet diaper for a few days. Maybe you've tried organic tampons but like a bad high school acquaintance, the pad will make her re-appearance into your life.

You will do anything not to wear pads including wearing and (staining) your underwear and wearing black pants (on light days) – praying you won't stain the seats. And just remember, while thongs and tampons are best friends, thongs and pads are enemies. Can you spell uncomfortable? Until it's proven otherwise, the only thing you want inside of you is a sperm producer (a.k.a your partner's thing), a transvaginal wand or your fertility doctor's (gloved) hand. You just hope your husband doesn't notice those red spotted underwear sitting in your laundry hamper.

"Millions of couples suffer from infertility, so why the f--k is everyone pregnant but me?" ~Infertile Naomi, Infertility Warrior

#33 The Infertile Answering Machine Message

Your mommy friend's answering machine goes something like this: *"Cara, Jack, Cindy, and Bobby can't come to the phone right now. We are too busy having fun as a family. Call us back!"* How incredibly sweet but totally boring. Yawn. If you are struggling with infertility, why not get creative with your answering machine message! Here are some suggestions:

- If you are calling to tell me that you're pregnant or having a baby shower, this line will
automatically disconnect. For all other calls, kindly leave a message after the beep.

- We can't come to the phone right now because my embryos are currently being removed from my ovaries and then transferred to a test tube. Leave a message!

- Susie, Jack and our little test tube can't come to the phone right now. We'll call you back after assisted hatching!

- Sorry we missed your call but it's ovulation time! We'll call you back in two days!

- I can't pick up the phone right now because I am too depressed about a negative pregnancy test. I'll call you back next month but only if my period is late.

- You've reached Martha on Monday morning. I am out of the office due to a transvaginal appointment but will return your call as soon as possible.

- I've stepped away from my desk to look for cervical mucus but will respond to your message immediately following my return.

- I will be late to the office every morning this week but I can't tell you why. Please leave a message. BEEP.

#34 Your Great Aunt Agnes is a Fertility Expert

Did you know that your mother, your great aunt Agnes and cousin Millie all became fertility specialists? When you weren't looking, they each got their diploma at the School of Bad Fertility Advice and graduated as an Infertility Expert. Apparently, they are now qualified to give you advice on a daily basis.

It seems that cousin Millie graduated top of her class and is now qualified to provide you excellent infertility advice such as 'just relax and it will happen' or 'drink this tea and you will get pregnant.' Mom also became an expert and has the right to question your decisions and fertility protocols. Her expert opinion including, *"my friend's daughter got pregnant after surgery for her blocked tube. You should try what she did,"* is great advice but probably not for someone with clear fallopian tubes. Thanks mother. I'll tell my doctor to book the unnecessary surgery.

And you're positive, eighty year old great aunt Agnes' advice that *"you only need one sperm"* will be taken into consideration during your next fertility procedure. Maybe your fertility doctor can invite Aunt Agnes into the procedure room for your next IVF cycle so she can help the doctor handpick the best sperm. It's also fantastic that your fertility expert sister-in-law thinks you should try Clomid even after your doctor said it wouldn't work for you. Maybe sister-in-law can write you an imaginary prescription on her fake doctors notepad.

Congratulations to the Fertility Advice Graduates! You are now qualified to give bad advice about infertility and also marriage, future children and careers.

#35 The Day Before Your Pregnancy Test

The day before your expected period is due is a beautiful day, filled with hope. Although you're quite sure there's no way you are actually pregnant, you have a tiny bit of hope left. This is the day when a pregnancy announcement can occur and you actually feel some happiness for them, instead of wanting to slit your wrists. After all, you might be pregnant too.

You feel like your period will come any second and you are experiencing all the classic fake pregnancy symptoms. Your left breast seems heavier than usual, your right nipple seems darker, and that pre-period headache hasn't arrived yet. You may just 'know' that you're not pregnant but you secretly have that bit of hope that you are.

You may run to the toilet every few minutes to check for redness or you may avoid the toilet altogether so you won't have to see the inevitable. The day of hope feels great and awful all in one. You just want to know but yet you don't want to know. Sometimes, you want to hold onto hope for just one day longer.

#36 You are Jealous of a Pregnant Dog

It's strange. You would never describe yourself as a jealous person. A woman could flirt with your husband and you're mildly flattered. Your friend gets a great promotion at work and you're genuinely happy for her. But when someone gets pregnant, whether a friend or a complete stranger, your jealous, evil side emerges.

It doesn't even matter who it is. You're completely envious of all your pregnant friends equally, but you are also jealous of complete strangers on the street; Facebook friends from your past; your mom's friend's daughter, and anyone else who happens to walk by you that looks pregnant. Good lord. You would even be jealous of a woman who got pregnant knowing that she suffered through years of fertility treatments. You would be jealous if your dog was having puppies, Peaches, the bird, got pregnant or even if a cartoon character was expecting. Damn you, Marge Simpson! You never had infertility problems with Bart, Lisa or Maggie! You were even envious of the Octomom. Wow. Bubbles, your goldfish, is having babies. Yup...Still jealous.

#37 The Infertile Birthday Wish

It's another birthday and it's time to blow out those candles. But golly gee wiz, what will you wish for? Duh! As you blow out your candles, you are convinced that every single person in that room knows what you wish for. Even your two year old nephew seems to know that you wish for a baby. Close your eye. Deep breath. *'By my next birthday, I wish to be pregnant or have a baby.'* Blow out those candles (all thirty-five of them!). The room is awkward as everyone claps politely, even your uterus applauds. How wonderful! She blew out all those candles but we all know what she wished for. *"I bet she wished for a baby,"* great aunt Greta whispers the obvious.

Oh great. Now, EVERYONE knows what you wished for, so how will it come true? Well maybe they are wrong! Maybe you actually wished for plentiful cervical mucus or for your husband to magically produce good quality semen! Not to worry, according to your fertility doctor you're still very young. You have plenty of time, right? Now, who wants another slice of fattening chocolate cake?

#38 You Had a Pregnancy Dream

During your two week wait, you tell yourself, 'self, if I'm pregnant, tell me in my dreams.' You fall asleep that night and hope your dreams tell you the answer. Unfortunately, you rarely dream about pregnancy. Instead, your nightly dreams are about your menstrual cycle, a negative pregnancy test or losing your baby. You often know your period is coming a week before simply because you dreamt it. Perhaps you had a dream that your period arrived and actor Tom Cruise handed you a tampon and said, *"you want the truth? You can't handle the truth!"* or something along those lines.

Once you dreamt that you took a pregnancy test but couldn't tell if it was two lines or just one. Those kind of dreams make you happy. Maybe your dream is trying to tell you that you're pregnant or perhaps it's trying to say, you may need to go to the eye doctors. You dream about other people having babies, so why is it never you own? 'Hey brain. Tonight can you please make me dream about having a positive pregnancy test?' Thank you in advance.

"If a tree falls in the forest, can anyone hear it? If an infertile bangs her head against the wall in a bathroom at a baby shower, can anyone hear her?" ~Infertile Naomi, Baby Shower Survivor

#39 Ways to Achieve a Positive Pregnancy Test

Do you always get a negative pregnancy test? Have you ever seen two lines on a pee stick? Here are some helpful ways to achieve your BFP (Big Fat Positive):

1. Draw on the second line yourself. Both marker and pen will work. Then show your husband the exciting news!

2. Cross your eyes until your sight becomes blurry and you actually see a second line.

3. Get a pregnant lady to pee on your stick.

4. Sneak into a pregnant lady's house and stick your pregnancy test in her leftover urine. Note: She may call the police so leave quickly.

5. Urinate following your HCG trigger shot (the hormone in the shot will actually produce two lines) and this will make you very happy.

6. Close your eyes when looking at the results and just assume it's positive.

7. Stick the pee test in a glass of apple juice. It's now a defective pregnancy stick! Return it to the store.

8. Pee on two sticks for two lines.

9. Ask a blind person to read you the results.

10. Try to buy the Octomom's old pregnancy test off eBay.

#40 Your Little Sister is Pregnant Before You

Hey baby sister, I'm so glad your uterus is working properly but can you hold off getting pregnant with baby number two until I get knocked up? You love your little sister, and you are truly happy that she didn't have fertility problems but seriously, you kind of wanted to provide the first grandchild. All those childhood years of fighting and what does she do? She gets pregnant before you can even say transvaginal wand. Maybe she even had one of those so-called accidental pregnancies or just tried one time and bing, bang, boom, it happened.

You have been trying for months and months and she sweeps in, looking all glowy and announces her pregnancy news. You are so happy for her (and only thirty to eighty percent jealous) but now she is talking about having another child! ARE YOU KIDDING? Two babies in two years? Is your husband's sperm made of magic? Do you lay the perfect grade A eggs? No fair! I'm telling mom on you!

Get ready for the family pregnancy announcement! Perhaps you're sitting at the family dinner table and see your sibling open her mouth slowly and see the words form: *"We haveeee something exciting to tellllll you."* In slow motion, you feel your chest start to cave in, your eyes start to tear and then you yearn to jump head first across the dining room table, land in your mother's homemade biscuits shouting, *"nooooooooo. Don't sayyyyyyy it."* But she says it (and you don't jump across the table); and everyone gets up to hug and celebrate. Because it is a wonderful celebration and sometimes, infertility makes you forget that. You tear up a bit, take a deep breath to blow out the negative energy, and look at your husband with a small but strong smile. You just know that one day it will be your turn too. Until then, you hold onto hope and just keep believing.

#41 You Know You're Having a Bad Infertile Day When...

You've had many bad infertile days. The 'wonderful' memory of crying on the bathroom floor at Pizza Hut; the time you had an emotional breakdown in the grocery store; and that magical moment when you cried in front of your boss. What wonderful memories. What freakin' wonderful infertile memories.

You also know it's a bad infertile day when...

1. Your boss asks you how you are today and you respond, *"emotionally unstable."*
2. Your waitress asks what type of eggs you want and you start telling her about your two beautiful fertilized embryos.
3. A telemarketer asks if you have children and you start telling him about your latest miscarriage.
4. You ask at the garden store if they have something to make you more fertile.
5. You burst into tears at Starbucks because the Barista asked if you wanted a kiddie-size hot chocolate.
6. You give the finger to a family of traveling ducks, crossing the street.
7. You tell the car salesman about your latest artificial insemination.
8. You curse a box of tampons at a visit to the drug store.
9. You have to wear a pirate patch so people can't see your swollen, tearful eyes.
10. You begin most conversations with a swear word.

#42 You Stopped Wearing Deodorant

Hey, what smells? Oh, it's you. In the world of infertility, you make up your own rules and somewhere along the way, you stopped wearing deodorant because you believe it affects your ability to get pregnant. Now, no one has ever told you this and you really have no concrete proof (other than what you read on Google, of course) but one day, you just stopped wearing it. Your armpits stink, and infertility has made you crazy. Sometimes you drink a special tea or eat a certain food or even refuse to get your eyebrows waxed because YOU believe that it affects your fertility. This week you decided that deodorant has got to go.

Perhaps you decided that your Lady Speed Stick penetrates into your armpit, travels down through your stomach to your uterus and produces an anti-fertility chemical. No medical professional has told you this but in your head, it makes logical sense.

Thank goodness you are not a doctor because all your patients would be eating pineapple cores, doing headstands, checking the toilet paper obsessively and looking at the color of their nipples on a daily basis.

#43 How to Find a Fertility Doctor

Here are some helpful tips on how to find a good fertility doctor:

1. Beware of a fertility doctor if their car license plate reads, 'The Octo Docto.'

2. Make sure the fertility clinic has good credentials. If their motto is, 'Wee Wee get you Pregnant,' you might want to try another clinic.

3. Check out the clinic's name. If it's called the 'Hump to Bump' or the 'Ute R US' clinic, please beware.

4. Make sure the doctor can pronounce fertility words correctly. You don't want a doctor who wants to increase your fat-ility, test your ovu-lactation or implant your umbrellas.

5. Beware of any doctor who shouts out *"hole in one!"* after an IUI.

6. Do not trust a doctor who refers to an IUI as a threesome.

7. If your fertility doctor asks you to feel her pregnant belly and invites you to her baby shower, you might want to see someone else.

8. You might wish to try another clinic should the women's bathroom also double as the semen analysis room.

9. Beware of any fertility doctor who says, *"we'll have you eating for eight in no time!"*

10. Leave the office if they have a sign on their door that reads, 'just relax and it will happen.'

"I wanted a perfect ending. Now I've learned, the hard way, that some poems don't rhyme, and some stories don't have a clear beginning, middle, and end. Life is about not knowing, having to change, taking the moment and making the best of it, without knowing what's going to happen next." ~Actress Gilda Radner

#44 You Stopped Drinking Coffee During Your Two Week Wait

Dear Coffee,

I love you. I'm so sorry we keep breaking up and then getting back together again month after month. The internet and fertility books advise me to limit your presence in my life but I still pine for you so much. One month, I will give you the silent treatment, refusing to even say hello to you in the morning. Another month, I will cheat on you with your less attractive and less tasty decaffeinated half cousin.

When I get a negative pregnancy test or Aunt Flow waves hello in my underpants, I return to you quickly like long lost lovers, embracing with cups and cups of caffeine love. The next moment, I may leave you again, running off with your tasteless nemesis, Tea-latte or Tea-ppuccino. But they just leave a bad after taste. I know it's okay we see each other in moderation but I still want you bad. Screw you fertility diet. Screw you!

I am forever your coffee lover.
xoxo

#45 You Are the Last One of Your Friends to Get Pregnant

And you were the first one to start trying! You wanted to be the first one of your friends to have a baby. Now, many months/years later, your friends have all gotten pregnant and some of them are even on baby number two. First Mindy-Jean got pregnant, then it was Molly-Sue, then Mary-Lou, and then very quickly, everyone in your circle of friends sported a baby bump.

Gee wiz, hasn't any of them ever heard of infertility before? Then, you had one childless couple left, but they soon announced a pregnancy too. Heck! Even all your virtual friends on Twitter have received their positives.

Feels bad, doesn't it? Not to worry, you are not the last one. Your co-worker, (the one with the PCOS-looking mustache), is not pregnant yet; and your little cousin, thankfully, isn't knocked up (although she is only fifteen years old). But just remember, even if you feel alone, you are never alone in infertility. There is help and support.

#46 You Are Not Pregnant During Your Dental Visit...Again

You measure your lack of pregnancies by that stupid dentist appointment. *'No Doctor Head Gear. I'm still not pregnant yet but thanks for asking.'* It begins with a routine trip to the dentist. You sit in the dental chair and think to yourself, *'the next time I sit in this dental chair, I will be pregnant.'* Six months later, you are back in the chair and still not pregnant. You may even ask the dentist politely if pregnant women are allowed teeth x-rays. *"We're not pregnant yet,"* you giggled nervously. *"But hopefully soon."* Suddenly you realized that you have been in that dentist chair dozens of times and you still aren't pregnant. That's a lot of un-pregnant dental cleanings.

Maybe the last time you sat in that chair you asked the dental hygienist if she could tell if you were pregnant by looking in your mouth (apparently pregnant women have bleeding gums. You learned this on the internet). But sadly, she says your gums are not bleeding.

You've had it. You are not going back to that dental chair unless you're pregnant. You don't care if your gums rot, you have eight cavities, you have to wear a full head and neck gear or you only have one tooth left, you WILL be pregnant next time you sit in that damn chair. Or you and your teeth are just not going back.

#47 The Best Places to Cry About Infertility

Infertility is great fun! One moment you feel sane and happy and the next, you're hormonal and crying in front of your boss. Once you start the infertility journey, you soon discover that you have frequent mental and emotional breakdowns. Perhaps, you are the type of person who is seemingly strong and put together but enter infertility, and you become an emotional wreck and a hormonal nightmare.

You are now able to cry on cue. You see a newborn baby in a restaurant – cue the tears. You walk into the toilet like a normal person who simply needs to pee. You step out of that toilet with tears running down your face and a maxi pad in your hand.

If you're going to have a weekly (or daily) emotional breakdown, why not choose some great crying locations! If Dave Letterman had a top ten reasons list of the best places to cry about infertility in public, they would be...

1. At your workplace. It's nice to attend meetings with tears streaming down your face.

2. On vacation. Tears and margaritas by the pool!

3. During your transvaginal wand appointment. Your fertility doctor might not even know you're sobbing because she is busy examining your other end.

4. At a baby shower. There are so many screaming children, no one will even hear your emotional sob fest in the guest of honor's bathroom.

5. In a public pool. Water and tears run down your face without notice and the chlorine will make your eyes turn red anyways.

6. In front of a maternity clothing store. People will just think you're a hormonal pregnant woman (just without the bump).

7. In a movie theater. It's dark and no one can see you.

8. Do the cry and drive. Pump up the music and start bawling!

9. At Walmart. The line-ups alone make everyone cry just a little.

10. When answering a call from a telemarketer. They will hang up on you quickly. Click.

#48 You Saw Your Fertility Doctor at a Restaurant

You are sitting at a nice restaurant, trying NOT to think about infertility, when all of a sudden you see someone who looks very familiar to you — *"Honey, isn't that our Reproductive Endocrinologist over at table seven?"*

It's sort of like when you were in school and saw one of your teachers out in public. You never actually realized that they existed outside of work. You simply believed that the fertility doctor, interns, vagina nurses and even the secretary (who takes all your money) just lived inside the clinic, and of all a sudden, your real world and (jealous, bitter) fertility world collide. You stare at this woman from across the room. You want to ask her a million questions but she probably doesn't want to talk about your vagina over her steak dinner.

Should you say hello? *Probably not.*
Should you ask her a question about ovulation while she eats her salad? *I don't think so.*
Should you chat with her about your hubby's low sperm count? *Maybe after she finishes her apple pie.*

Perhaps she could tell you if you're pregnant right there in the fancy restaurant. Sounds like an appropriate dinner conversation. After all, this woman looks into your vagina on a weekly basis, she should be your personal on-call doctor. Instead, you don't make eye contact with your doctor, and go back to your happy place where fertility doctors and nurses all live within the clinic and their sole purpose in life is getting you pregnant.

"Our greatest glory is not in failure but in rising up every time we fail."
~Ralph Waldo Emerson

#49 You Keep Staining Your Underwear Because You Won't Buy Pads

Once you've joined the 'Infertility Club,' you also get an honorary membership to the 'Soiled Underwear Club' too….. Congratulations? You suffer from period pantie denial (PPD). Every month, you go through a mild state of denial, refusing to pre-purchase tampons or those (extremely uncomfortable and disgusting) pads which ALWAYS leads to underwear that has been…well… soiled. The longer you go through infertility, the longer you are plagued by PPD. You may even have a few 'period panties' (PP), saved just for your monthly occasions. You start wearing those PP when you feel your period is imminent or refuse to wear them, subconsciously believing that this month will be your month. And when your period does arrive, you slip on a pair of pre-stained underwear and sit in your own filth.

No doubt, you don't want your husband to witness your fabulous period panties. He might not find them as sexy as the thongs you use to wear when you were first dating. Now, those Walmart PP are covered with colorful red and brown spots and a splatter of artistic drips.
"Honey, don't look in the laundry this month. My underwear has been soiled again." You are a proud infertile, and President and CEO of the Soiled Underwear Club.

#50 Ways to Drive an Infertile Crazy

We are hormonal, pregnancy-obsessed, baby bump envious, addicted to fertility drugs, a tad crazy at times but lovable all the same! But (somewhere) underneath the hysterical sobbing and emotional breakdowns, we still keep our sense of humor.

Here are some insider tips on ways to annoy an infertile:

1. Tell us how you got pregnant on your first try and then complain about your pregnancy symptoms.

2. Ask us to take weekly photos of your pregnancy belly and post them on Facebook.

3. When we come to your house, stain all of your toilet paper bright red.

4. Playfully hide our time-sensitive fertility medication.

5. Tell us that our fertility clinic telephoned but you can't remember the message.

6. Tell us a story about someone you know who adopted and then suddenly got pregnant.

7. Tell us to relax and stop trying so it will just happen.

8. Use the acronym 'BFN' when referring to your cousin, <u>B</u>illy <u>F</u>. <u>N</u>ewman.

9. Complain about your children, daily.

10. Ask us to pick up some diapers and baby products for you.

11. Wait until the first day of our period and then ask us to help plan your baby shower.

12. Tell us that you accidentally spilled our fertility medication into the toilet.

13. Remind us how old we are and how we still don't have children.

14. Ask us if we're pregnant yet.

#51 Your Life is an Infertile Soap Opera

Ever feel like your life is a soap opera? You feel like you have a secret infertile self that you hide from others, filled with drama, emotion, heartache, hope and an insane amount of sex. Yes, you're living an infertile soap opera, just without the accidental pregnancy, an embryo switch, and a bartender named Chase who may or may not be your baby daddy.

The Young and the Tender Breastless
Plot: Dominique is in her two week wait after an emotional embryo transfer. She feels rage at her doctor for telling her that she is 'still young' and has plenty of time to get pregnant. She continues to examine her breasts for early pregnancy symptoms.

All my (Test Tube) Children: Olivia and Tanner want a baby but a twisted fallopian tube, a misshapen uterus, poor egg quality and low sperm motility stand in their way.

The Cold and the Beautiful: Cricket and her husband, Braden, get into another fight about her obsession with wanting a child. He disagrees with her idea that they should just steal a baby.

As your Insides Churn: Victoria is filled with heartache after her little sister announces she's pregnant. Selena gets her period during her friend's baby shower. Tiffany-Melinda bursts into tears after her mother-in-law emails her another article about how to increase her fertility.

Days of our Hives: Harlowe is rushed to the hospital after suffering from an allergic reaction from her fertility medication. Devastatingly, the doctor also discovers she is suffering from OHSS and her embryo transfer has been canceled.

General (Fertility) Hospital: Tad discovers that his lover, Summer, is having an affair with her fertility doctor and a transvaginal wand.

One Life to Live: Corrina and her (seemingly) loving husband, Prescott, feel like if they only have one life to live, it sure as hell better be a fertile one!

#52 Your First Thought After Hearing Someone is Pregnant

When you find out someone is pregnant, a normal first reaction is, *"wow. Congratulations! That is great news. I'm so happy for you!"* But you're an infertile and that's typically not your first reaction, even if you don't want to admit it.

YOUR DAD: *"Cousin Martha just called. She is pregnant! Isn't that great news!"*

What you automatically think:

- Are you kidding me? Martha just got married.
- How many people are going to get pregnant before it's our turn already!
- Great. Now everyone is pregnant but me.
- But we started trying long before she did.
- What the fertile! She's still so bloody young.
- What the fertile! She's still in school and he has no money.
- Wow. He really must have super sperm to get her pregnant so quickly.
- Good for her.*
- So, who cares? Why are you telling me this?*

*Note: You will tend to have a more bitter and envious reaction should a pregnancy announcement occur during your period or following a failed cycle and negative pregnancy test.

YOUR ACTUAL RESPONSE: *"That's great news, dad. Pass along my congratulations. I'm so happy for them."*

You respond this way because it's not socially acceptable to become a raging infertile lunatic in public. Because you are strong and you refuse to show anyone your jealous and bitter side. Because you know it's actually good news even if it doesn't feel that way. Because one day it will be your turn too. You respond this way because you are awesome and strong and fantastic, even if you don't always remember that.

#53 You Order Infertility Movies From the Library

For the last two weeks, you have been trying to find the movie, Mother and Child, at your local library. Why? Because you heard it's a really good movie? No. Because the movie has to do with infertility.

It happens like this. You see a movie trailer, whether a comedy or drama, where the main character is struggling with infertility, adopting or yearning for a child and you have to see it. It doesn't matter if it's a comedy about Jennifer Lopez getting pregnant after an IUI or Jennifer Aniston looking for a sperm donor by her fortieth birthday. You want to see this movie because you like to torture yourself.

Some people claim they have 'gay-dar.' When it comes to movies, you have infertility-dar and preg-dar. You end up seeing a movie, leaving the theater in tears and feeling angry that they didn't portray infertility in a realistic light. *What the fertile?!* Jennifer Lopez got pregnant on her first IUI? What happened to doing multiple IUIs and then moving onto IVF? And how come Jennifer Aniston finds a sperm donor and she suddenly becomes pregnant? And of course, you also cried a little during the ridiculous comedy, Baby Mama, where Tina Fey wants to be a baby mama but needs some help. Word of caution. When you see a movie with an infertility plot, it usually has a happy baby ending.

But since you never learn, for the last two weeks, you have been to four libraries trying to reserve the movie, Mother and Child. And this time, you will make your husband watch it with you so you can torture him as well. Until the next infertility movie trailer and the film/torture cycle begins again.

"Perseverance is failing 19 times and succeeding the 20th." ~Actress Julie Andrews

#54 Bootcamp for New Infertiles

Dear Infertility Virgin,

Welcome to the club! As a seasoned infertile, we would like to pass along a few pieces of wisdom as you start your (extremely long) journey towards parenthood.

Start trying on your wedding night. What? You and your partner are not ready yet? Who cares! After your twentieth BFN, you'll wish you started trying on your first date.

See a specialist after one month of trying. Most medical professionals will tell you to try naturally for one year before seeing a specialist. They got that wrong. You'll try for one month, then another, then another and then you'll have to wait a few months until you can get an appointment with your doctor. By that time, it's almost a year anyways. Be proactive.

You will do strange things to enhance your fertility. You will read many books on how to get pregnant and you'll try strange things including a full headstand after intercourse and eating pineapple in excess during your two week wait.

You will soon know what cervical mucus looks like. Never heard of ovulation or cervical mucus before? You are about to become an expert and graduate of Cervical Mucus Academy. You will soon know how to spell 'Intrauterine Insemination' and all those other long spelling fertility words.

You will cry in random places after getting your period. You will go into a bathroom stall completely normal and leave in tears. Don't be surprised if you have emotional breakdowns in public and in front of your boss. If you're going to sob, don't forget to pick your favorite designated crying area and bring some tissues.

Your mother will clip out articles about infertility for you. Some articles will be useful but most will just make you want to cry. Continue to love your mother but don't read all the articles.

You will be jealous of anything that gets pregnant. It won't matter if it's a pregnant dog, cat, fish or Barbie Doll, when someone (or something) gets pregnant before you, you will feel jealous. And then you will pretend that you aren't.

It will feel like everyone on Facebook is pregnant. Facebook will soon feel like Fertilitybook, where everyone is pregnant or has two kids.

You will examine the toilet paper often. Each time you go to the toilet, you will examine that toilet paper for signs of your period. It will soon become impossible not to look at the toilet paper.

If you relax, it still won't happen. You could send your uterus on a vacation and chances are, it will come home tanned but still not pregnant.

Don't give up. Be determine and keep believing. One day, it will be your turn too.

#55 What Not to Say to Your Fertility-Challenged Wife

Honey, I love you but sometimes I need a little extra support from you. Here are some suggestions of what NOT to say to your fertility-challenge spouse:

1. It's a buddy's fishing weekend so I might have to miss your ovulation period this month.
2. Both my ex-girlfriends are pregnant.
3. They had a sale on red-colored toilet paper so I bought some.
4. Your basal thermometer accidentally fell into the toilet.
5. The fertility clinic called with your test results but I accidentally deleted the message.
6. My sister and her boyfriend of three months are pregnant.
7. Can we use a condom this month?
8. You look bloated. Are you getting your period?
9. Do we have to? I'm not in the mood tonight.
10. I don't know what's the rush. We're still young.
11. I told my sister you would be happy to plan her baby shower.
12. Why are you crying? It's only a period.
13. Do I really have to do another semen test? It's so much work!
14. I'd come with you to your fertility appointment but it's so early in the morning and I like to sleep in.
15. Did you gain weight this cycle?
16. I forgot to put your fertility medication in the refrigerator.

17. I heard if we just relax, it might happen.
18. I know we're saving for IVF but I bought this really awesome video game.
19. Oops! I accidentally injected your needle in the wrong spot.
20. I know I was suppose to remind you to take your HCG shot at exactly 10pm but there was this really funny movie on TV.
21. You have a lot of zits on your forehead.
22. Sorry about missing the cup during our IUI.
23. My co-worker got pregnant after adopting.
24. I told my sister you'd take her shopping at the maternity store.
25. Check out my ex-girlfriend's cute belly photos on Facebook!
26. I don't think your breasts look any bigger.
27. My friend's wife needed some pregnancy sticks so I gave her your supply.
28. I accidentally switched your folic acid vitamins with your old birth control pills.
29. Are you crying AGAIN?
30. Angelina and Brad are pregnant with triplets. Isn't that great?
31. I think you're too obsessed with infertility.
32. I think we should wait a little longer before seeing a fertility specialist.
33. I know you're upset about getting your period today but I invited my friend and his pregnant wife over for dinner.
34. Don't worry hun, we'll get pregnant next month.
35. Why do we always have to talk about getting pregnant?
36. I want to switch back to wearing briefs instead of boxer shorts.
37. I invited your mother to our fertility counseling session.
38. What's a two week wait?
39. I got us two free tickets to the Baby Show Expo! Want to go?
40. I invited my mother to your embryo retrieval procedure.
41. I know you bought that pineapple for yourself but I ate it all.
42. No. I definitely don't see two lines.
43. There, there dear. It's only a period.
44. You wouldn't look good as a pregnant woman anyways.
45. Can you postpone our IUI until Saturday? Thursday isn't good for me.

#56 You Refuse to Book a Vacation During a Fertility Cycle

Last week your sweet husband innocently said to you, *"honey, let's book a vacation in February."* Your first thought: How can we book a vacation that far in advance? I know it's six months away but what if we're in the middle of fertility treatments? Don't we have to save money anyways? What if I'm pregnant by then? I probably won't want to fly during first trimester.

What you actually say to him: *"That sounds nice, dear* (except you don't usually call him dear.
You aren't seventy years old). *Let's just book it closer to the time."* It's best to keep those infertile thoughts to yourself. It will also save you the following argument:

Him: *"I'm tired of having my life revolve around fertility treatments! Can't we just book a vacation for once!"*

You: (tears) *"You don't understand! Everyone has a baby but us"* (storm upstairs to the bedroom. Slam door).
Fertility Tip: If you are having some crazy infertile thoughts, it's best to keep them to yourself.

#57 Everyone at Walmart is Pregnant

Welcome to Walmart. The store where everyone is pregnant. That sixteen year old cashier is pregnant. The lady in aisle five is pregnant. That woman in the pickle aisle is pregnant. You can no longer go into a Walmart without running into someone who is (a) pregnant, or (b) has at least five children. And it's not just the customers. All the employees are pregnant too. The door greeter, (who looks like she's eighty years old), appears to have a baby bump. The cashier, who looks like she could be on the reality show, Sixteen and Pregnant, is expecting. It's like you have to be pregnant in order to work there. To make things worse, Walmart once introduced Midge, Barbie's pregnant friend, in the toy department. Sure. Barbie's doll friend can get pregnant but you are still stuck in the infertile aisle.

ATTENTION WALMART SHOPPERS! IF YOU ARE INFERTILE, PLEASE LEAVE THE STORE IMMEDIATELY!

#58 Ten Things You Should Never Say to Your Childless Friend

1. I heard about this lady who got implanted with the wrong embryo. Did that happen at your fertility clinic? The thought has crossed your mind a million times that your clinic could implant the wrong sperm or egg. After all, your little eggies and his slow-moving sperm are outside your body and hanging out in a lab room. You've heard stories where a fertility doctor was sued because she implanted the wrong embryo into the wrong uterus. But unless your future baby comes out a completely different color, speaks a foreign language or looks exactly like the other couple doing IVF at the same time as you, then you're keeping the baby. Hell, you'll keep the baby regardless.

2. You can have one of my eggs! First of all, thank you for the pretend offer. If you really mean it, then you will be happy to inject yourself with fertility drugs for the next four to six weeks, feel swollen and bloated, and later retrieve your eggs under general anesthesia. Thank you but I'd rather use my own, more attractive DNA. Thanks again for the pretend offer but I'll pass.

3. We relaxed and it just happened! Neat-o, for you! I'll ask my doctor if relaxing will improve my disgruntled uterus, my lack of fallopian tubes and my rapidly maturing eggs.

4. I am going to announce my pregnancy at your birthday party next week! Tell me right before you are going to make your announcement and I'll smash the cake in your face. The photos will be priceless!

5. Did you ever try Clomid? Do you even know what Clomid is? Even though my fertility doctor doesn't recommend it, if you can tell me what Clomid is used for, then I'll take it.

6. My cousin's neighbor's friend's hair dresser did IVF. Do you want her phone number? Sure. I'd love to call up a complete stranger and talk about my personal fertility issues. (Ring, Ring. Hello? Hi. You don't know me but I got your number from someone I don't know either. My husband has low sperm motility and we are going through IVF right now. Want to chat about it over coffee and folic acid?).

7. I found your fertility medication in the fridge and I accidentally threw it in the garbage. Is that a problem? I found a wad of one hundred dollar bills in your wallet and did the same. Is that a problem?

8. Do you want to come salsa dancing after your IUI procedure? During my two week wait, I don't want to shake my belly or move my body at all. I would like to stay still for exactly ten days straight whether it's logical or not.

9. You don't look pregnant. Never tell an infertile that she doesn't look pregnant. She wants to be pregnant. She wants to look pregnant. She wants to feel that she could be pregnant. Telling her she looks a bit fat this month will make her happy.

10. When I was your age, I had four children by now. That's just wonderful, Great Aunt Gerta, but I wouldn't be so proud of yourself. Your children didn't turn out that great. Debbie had a kid at fourteen years old; Patsy married her first cousin; Billy-Bob won a hot dog eating contest, and isn't Lenny a full-time juggler? Again, congratulations on procreating.

"Please, on Mother's Day, have some compassion. If you see someone without kids, do not ask them why they don't have children, why they don't just adopt, or if they are pregnant. Please be kind. Be quiet and pass the dip." ~Actress Nia Vardalos

#59 You have a Fertility Appointment on Mother's Day

What are you doing this Mother's Day? A nice brunch? A spa day out with mom? Nope. You will be putting your legs up in stirrups and enjoying a transvaginal wand appointment. No doubt, you are dreading Mother's Day (also recognized as National Infertiles Worst Nightmare Day). This is the day where all your mommy friends will be posting photos of their Mother's Day on Facebook, and every status update will say, 'Cherish being a Mother today.' Blah.

Ironically, you will probably have a fertility appointment scheduled on this day. While little kids everywhere are making breakfast in bed for their fertile mother, you will be waking up at six in the morning to drive to your blood and ultrasound appointment, change into a blue gown and sit with the other non-moms while you wait your turn for a fertility doctor to poke around your vagina.

"Right side. There is a 1.1 follicle, 1.4 follicle, 0.3 follicle. Left side is quiet," your fertility doctor will say. Damn you, transvaginal wand. Maybe I should make you breakfast in bed! Perhaps you will have an IUI, embryo retrieval or transfer scheduled on this day. That way, you will probably miss out on taking your own mother out for brunch. *"Sorry mom. Gotta miss Mother's Day again this year. We're getting artificially inseminated."* Doesn't Hallmark make a greeting card for that occasion? You WILL survive Mother's Day. You WILL get through it. You are a mother too. You just haven't met your baby yet.

#60 Infertility Myths

MYTH: Your fertility clinic will never call you back
It might feel like they will never call you back but eventually your fertility clinic will call. You have left a voice message for your clinic early this morning. You could be calling for any number of reasons including (but not limited to), your pregnancy test results, IVF fertilization report, an inquiry about ovulation or some embarrassing question about spotting and if that's normal. *"Hi. It's Infertile calling again. I went for my beta blood test this morning. Please give me a call*

back with the results." You called them at 8:30am. 9am, no phone call. 10am, no phone call. 10:15am, check to see if phone is working. It is. 11am, no phone call. 11:15am, phone rings and it's your mother. You quickly hang up on her. As you wait for the call, the phone comes with you into the bathroom and you contemplate calling them again.

FOR THE LOVE OF INFERTILITY, WHY WON'T THEY CALL ME BACK?
You start thinking that it must be bad news or you would have heard from them sooner. You wait by the phone the entire day until the clinic finally calls you back at 4:59pm. See, they do call back.

MYTH: You will get pregnant before your little sister
False! Even though you got married first, started trying for a baby first and you are five years older, your little sister will, most likely, get pregnant before your uterus can even say, *"what the fertile?"* Your sweet little sister, Janie, will likely do one of two things, (a) get married and come back from her honeymoon pregnant, or (b) announce that she got pregnant accidentally. Not only will she get pregnant first, she will also conceive baby number two before your next IUI. Congratulations to Janie.

MYTH: You would be thrilled to plan your sister-in-law's baby shower
OMG! Your sister-in-law, Fertile Franny, is pregnant…again! You found out on Facebook when she posted her twelve week ultrasound photo. Isn't that like her fifth baby already? She expects you to plan her baby shower and you would be absolutely thrilled to be the hostess. FALSE. You put on a fake smile and say, *"of course, I'd love to plan your shower."* Then, you politely run to the bathroom where you spend the next twenty minutes sobbing on the toilet seat. You don't want to go to her shower, let alone plan it. In actuality, you would rather not attend any baby showers, first birthday parties or family events where babies and preggos are invited. But you will put on that false smile, bake little blue and pink cupcakes and throw Franny one hell of a baby shower. Fertility Tip: Just try not to spike the punch.

MYTH: Breaking a negative pregnancy stick in half won't make you feel better
Yes, It will. It also helps to place the stick on your driveway, get in your car and drive over that negative pregnancy stick until it makes you feel better.

#61 You Refuse to See Your Friend Until You Get Pregnant

You have a friend that you see once a month for lunch. You now have a monthly lunch date reminder that you still aren't pregnant yet.

January Lunch: *"How are things? Are you pregnant yet?"*
February Lunch: *"How are you guys? I was hoping you'd have a baby bump by now."*
March Lunch: *"Really? Still not pregnant? I swore you'd be pregnant this time."*
April Lunch: Cancelled!

The last time you made lunch plans with your friend, you swore to yourself that you would never schedule another lunch date with her until you were pregnant. It's really too bad because you like her a lot, and it's not like you can explain this to her.

"Yeah, Sorry, Melinda but we can no longer see each other until I'm pregnant. Don't worry, I'm sure we'll see each other sometime between next month and the year 2025."

And you realize this is not a rational solution but somewhere over cob salad and your second glass of wine, you decide that you are willing to put the friendship on hold for a few more months. Having lunch with her is sort of like visiting the dentist anyways. Every time you visit the dentist you think, *'next time I visit the dentist, I will be pregnant.'* But next time comes and goes and you are forced to have those darn pregnancy no-no x-rays and provide the dental hygienist with a list of your current fertility medications. Sorry Melinda! But lunch has been canceled. Indefinitely. We will renew the friendship at a later fertile date.

#62 It's Great to be Infertile Because...

So what if your uterus isn't behaving! Who cares if your husband's sperm has more tails than a dog! Don't feel sorry for us! There are lots of positive aspects to being (temporarily) infertile such as:

1. No awkward sex talk to your future children! Explaining the birds and the bees to the children will be fun! *"Little Tommy, when a mommy and a daddy love each other, they drive to a fertility clinic and four years later, you are conceived with a lot of love and a little test tube."*

2. By the time you are pregnant, your friends are already finished having kids. You can borrow all of their baby stuff (even if they are stained with poop and vomit).

3. During IVF or IUI, your partner doesn't even have to be present during conception! Just send him a quick text once it's done. *"Honey, we did it! How was it for you?"*

4. When you go to sleep at night, you still get to sleep through the night (although you may wake up during the night to cry about infertility).

5. You get to cry about infertility in random places. Why go to a boring old grocery store just to shop? Yawn. Boring. Having an emotional breakdown in the tampon aisle, now that's interesting!

6. Your friends all offer to let you have their bratty kids. Great! So don't call the police when we actually try to keep them. We have a verbal agreement.

7. When your quintuplets arrive, you'll get your own reality show called, IVF Mama Plus Five!

8. You get to have surgery to help improve your fertility. The positive side? Time off work and the hospital offers these delicious pudding cups for lunch! Lip-smacking!

9. Your mommy friend have stretch marks, sagging breasts and wrinkles. You only have weight gain and acne due to fertility medication.

10. Whoever said infertility was terrible obviously never met your hot fertility doctor! He can inseminate you anytime!

Even if it doesn't always feel this way and you think you will never get pregnant, infertility is,
most likely, temporary. Hope and determination are permanent.

#63 Infertility: The Movie

If your infertile life was a movie, it would be called…

Category: Suspense
Whodunit? I just murdered my period.
My husband has a business trip during my ovulation dates and I'm going to kill his boss.

I waited by the phone all day for my fertility clinic to call me back.
Will she ever find a pair of underwear that isn't stained red?

Romance
(Over) Eat, Pray, No Glove.
I have a bottle of wine and fertility drugs in the fridge.
The IVF Story: We made a baby and my husband wasn't even in the room.

Dark Comedy
My husband has low sperm count and other great stories.
I can't afford fertility treatment but I can afford this bottle of alcohol.
I'm home on a Saturday night crying about infertility.
I once took a pregnancy test in the bathroom at a flea market.
My husband is not allowed in a whirlpool until we conceive.
My hubby may have low sperm motility but he sure is sexy!

Western
I'm ovulating, cowboy. Giddy Up!

Inspirational
My period is three hours late and I feel giddy.
My eggs might be cracked but my heart is still hopeful.
The Facebook Story: I just deleted all my pregnant friends.
I might be old and grey before I conceive, but it will happen.

"Hope never abandons you, you abandon it." ~George Weinberg

#64 Your Mommy Friends Left Your New Year's Eve Party at 7pm

Your crazy, wild New Year's Eve party. The booze. The dancing. The countdown to midnight. Unfortunately, none of those things happened because your friends and their children left the party at 7pm. You invited your (fertile) friends over for a wild New Year's Eve bash at your house.

You sent out an email invitation and received the immediate replies:

- We'll be there after nap time!
- We're ready to party! But no booze for us. I'm breastfeeding and tired so my husband will be the designated driver.
- Can't wait! Can you make sure that everything you serve is nut-free?
- We'll have to leave early though because I'm pregnant and can't stay up until midnight.

Your guests arrived promptly. Missy brings a nut-free cake and a bag of toys for her kids and Sally-Ann brings a bouncy chair for her baby. Steven 'I-use-to-get-drunk-at-every-party' is now sipping on water and burping a baby. There are poopie diapers in your garbage and breast milk in your fridge (right next to your fertility medication). Little Tommy lost a ball under your couch, and someone is talking about baby Sophie's constipation problems. My God! She hasn't pooped since last Sunday!

You bought seven bottles of wine and only one got opened. No one touched the raw sushi because most of your friends are pregnant; and Betsy is breastfeeding on your bed. Dinner ends quickly and everyone leaves before 7:00pm. Let the prolonged countdown to midnight begin. Five hours to midnight...Happy New Year!

#65 Surviving an Infertile Halloween

This time last year, you were starting your first IUI. So how come a full year later, you are no closer to a pregnancy?
Here are some tips on surviving another infertile Halloween.

1. Dress snazzy this Halloween! Dress up as a bottle of folic acid, a broken uterus, a negative pregnancy test or an
8.2 celled embryo (Note: not all costumes are available at Walmart).

2. When kids ring your doorbell, resist the urge to keep them. Stealing a child is wrong.

3. Answer the door sobbing and tell the first kid you see about your last failed cycle.

4. Rent a scary movie about the childless couple and her rapidly deteriorating eggs.

5. Give out raisins for Halloween. Eat all the chocolate yourself because you deserve it.

6. Leave a note on the door that says, '*sorry kids. No Halloween candy here because I'm ovulating tonight!*'

7. Put on a beard and tell everyone you're dressed as a woman with PCOS.

8. If anyone in your office dresses up as a pregnant woman, mention to your boss that she asked to work overtime this week.

9. Go to your morning fertility appointment dressed as a positive pregnancy test.

10. Answer the door with a smile on your face and hope in your heart. You may not be pregnant this Halloween but one day, you will take your future children out trick or treating. Only an infertile could despise a holiday that is dedicated to chocolate, candy and sugar. Eat up!

#66 Discovering You Just Got Your Period

Step 1: Expect arrival of your period.

Step 2: Check toilet paper hourly.

Step 3: Feel slightly hopeful when your period is thirty minutes late.

Step 4: Keep checking toilet paper hourly.

Step 5: Light spotting.

Step 6: Insert swear word.

Step 7: Begin crying on the toilet seat.

Step 8: Random thoughts include: Is this really my period or is it implantation bleeding?

Step 9: You still remain 1% hopeful but you just know it's over.

Step 10: Check toilet paper again.

Step 11: Bleeding gets heavier. Infertile sobbing and runny nose begins.

Step 12: You don't have any pads because you refused to buy them. Run to store.

Step 13: Take a pregnancy test, just in case. Swear a lot when it comes out negative.

Step 14: More tears and increased moodiness begins. Husband/partner doesn't understand why
you're crying on the toilet seat.

Step 15: Call fertility clinic and sob into the phone… *"Hi, it's Infertile* (insert your name). *I'm calling again on my Day One…."*

Step 16: Screw you, folic acid pills. You are not taking any this week.

Step 17: Buy a large cup of caffeinated coffee, chocolate and a bottle of wine. Enjoy.
Repeat next month.

The Period. Punctuation for the end but also meaning a new beginning and starting fresh.

#67 Infertility Urban Legends

Having sex leads to pregnancy. Having intercourse to get pregnant? How is that even possible?

Having sex during ovulation increases your chance of getting pregnant. You've had sex before, during and after ovulation so where's the baby?

Fertiles have baby showers to celebrate the upcoming birth of their child. Untrue. The baby shower was created to torture infertiles.

Facebook was developed as a new way to connect with your friends. In reality, founder Mark Zuckerberg created Facebook so fertiles can post ultrasound photos, belly shots and further torture infertiles.

The fertility clinic helps to get people pregnant. In reality, if you see a pregnant woman at your fertility clinic, she is probably a paid actress to make it seem like couples are actually getting pregnant.

If you relax, you will get pregnant. Untrue. You'll conceive when you're stressed out.

You only need one egg and one sperm. You've had multiple eggs and millions of sperm which only resulted in the conception of a large bottle of wine and a box of chocolates.

#68 The TV Show: Infertiles Got Talent

Ever watch that reality show, America's Got Talent? Contestants with (and without) talent showcase their stuff on a TV reality show. We beg to differ. Infertiles are the ones with talent.
Vote for us! Here are some of our special talents:

- Only an infertile could have timed intercourse and then do a full gymnastic headstand for
thirty minutes.

- Only an infertile could hold in their pee after drinking a liter of water for an embryo transfer.

- Only an infertile could wake up at 6am, go to the fertility clinic at 7am and still make it to her

morning meeting by 9.

- Only an infertile could take Clomid, have side effects and still ace her client presentation.

- Only an infertile could hold up a pregnancy test in a dimly lit bathroom, trying to find the
second line.

- Only an infertile could fake an award-winning smile after hearing a pregnancy announcement.

- Only an infertile could buy cough syrup because she heard it helps increase her ovulation fluid.

- Only an infertile knows exactly what cervical mucus looks and feels like.

- Only an infertile could pre-fail a cycle before it even happened yet.

- Only an infertile could give an opera-like sob after getting her period in a public bathroom.

- Only an infertile could be such a strong person who refuses to give up because she knows one
day, it WILL happen.

"Don't let infertility knock you down... Let it knock you up instead!"
~Infertile Naomi, Professional Toilet Paper Examiner

#69 There Must Be Something in the Water

Eleven of your co-workers are pregnant. Mindy from Accounting is pregnant; Kelly-Sue from HR is expecting and even Bob and his partner Jimbo are having a baby via surrogate. *"There must be something in the water,"* your co-workers say. *"You will be next!"* Seriously? You've been drinking the same water from the same water cooler for months and you're still not pregnant yet. And you highly doubt that Bob and Jimbo's surrogate strolled over to your office and had a glass before she magically got pregnant (on the first attempt, of course). Listen up, co-workers! There is nothing in the water! You know because you foolishly convinced yourself that maybe some type of pregnancy hormone was actually lurking in the water, and you've been drinking bottle after bottle (also making your co-workers suspicious because you've been peeing so much too).

You know what is actually in the water?
Arsenic
Calcium
Selenium
Cadmium
Chromium
Mercury
Nitrate
and perhaps some delicious lead.

So unless your fertilized egg and a fertility doctor is swimming around inside that water cooler, there is nothing in the water that made your whole office pregnant. Perhaps that Linda from sales and marketing is just a tad slutty. Just saying.

#70 Trying For a Baby Is So Much Fun!

Yes. Great Aunt Gertie. You're right. Trying for a baby is FUN! But by FUN do you mean...

...Having routine timed intercourse with your great nephew for months on end, and then elevating my legs to help his boys swim upstream; sticking a pink thermometer in my mouth each morning and then charting my basal temperature? How about when I examine the toilet paper obsessively; drink raspberry leaf tea; and stick needles between my eyes and in my belly while an acupuncturist named Felicity tells me to relax. Yes, trying for a baby is definitely a great time. Just ask my husband when he had to provide a semen analysis test on nine different occasions and then had to chat about it openly with a strange doctor. It was also a blast during my HSG fertility test; and when we had to talk to a fertility intern named Camille about our sex life. I would also say it was good times during all those early morning transvaginal wand appointments; and following our seventh failed IUI when I sobbed on the bathroom toilet. It was also quite enjoyable when I had to miss work meetings because I was having eggs removed from my ovaries; when all my friends got pregnant before me; and when I gained excess weight from those super fun fertility drugs.

But yes, Aunt Gertie, you are completely right. Trying for a baby is fun but sometimes it's also a bit…what's the word?…..Trying.

#71 You Have Already Named Your Children

When most women get pregnant, she spends the next nine months trying to think of a suitable name for her child. Great news! You are not like most women. The infertile woman has already chosen her child's name long before she tried to conceive. You had a lot time to think about baby names or who you wanted to name your child after. You have spent hours asking your husband if he likes the name Mack or if he would be interested in having a daughter named Clomid. Either way, you know your future children's names. But what if someone inadvertently steals your name?

You've been trying to conceive the longest which should mean that no one should have the right to take your names. You picked them out long before your BFF even started trying! Stealing is against the law and should not be taken lightly. A lawyer would advise you to send out a written document to all your fertile friends and family indicating your confirmed or potential baby name choices. Please inform them that these names are now off limits for any future children but you will consider special circumstances, if asked prior to delivery. If the couple conceives on the first try, all names must be forwarded to you for approval. You have the right to dismiss any names at any time or any reason. This written agreement will, most likely, hold up in a court of law.

#72 Your Friends Stop Asking if You are Pregnant

The F word. Fertility, that is. A word you don't often say in public but you'll yell to your husband at least once a week. Fertility You!

When you first started trying, you found support in your friends. They would ask about your fertility problems and give you a shoulder to cry on. But one by one, they got bit by the stork and you started confiding in them less and less. Then, they became afraid to talk to you about it. The truth is you don't mind talking about it (but it really depends on the day), and they seem very afraid to bring up the F word. You both now talk around it. When you get together, they cautiously hint at topics about infertility but will rarely bring it up directly. In fact, they now speak to you in code.

"I heard your cousin is pregnant" this means *"are you pregnant yet?"*
"How are things?" – this means *" are you pregnant yet?"*
"Did you see that new movie about adoption?" this means *"are you pregnant yet?"*

Your friends mean well, they really do, and you can tell they are really trying to be sensitive about your situation. But sometimes they should just blurt out, *"IT'S BEEN FIVE YEARS ALREADY, WHY IN THE WORLD AREN'T YOU PREGNANT YET? WHAT IS WRONG WITH YOU?"* I'm sure that will make you both feel better. Clearly.

#73 The Real Ways to Enhance Your Fertility

As a veteran infertile, you already know that there are many ways to enhance your fertility including:

1. Getting regular exercise.
2. Taking folic acid.
3. Avoiding artificial lubricants.
4. Having intercourse during your ovulation days.
5. Reducing caffeine and alcohol.
6. Relaxing.
7. Keeping his parts nice and cool.
8. Assuming the right position.
9. Charting your temperature.
10. Doing it every forty eight hours if his sperm count is low.

…Blah, Blah, Blah. BORING!

You have tried all of these ways but nothing seems to work. You're no doctor, but perhaps you've been getting the wrong advice about how to increase your fertility. Here are some better ways to enhance your fertility:

1. Do it in a public place, preferably under an apple tree.
2. Before intercourse, take a piece of broccoli and swallow whole.
3. Do a full handstand after intercourse, followed by a back flip. Your husband's applause will increase his sperm count.
4. Eat a bowl of melted chocolate without a spoon following intercourse.
5. Have intercourse before watching Oprah but never during Dr. Phil.
6. Create a fertility dance to a Paula Abdul song (other artists won't be as effective).
7. Do a fertility dance at midnight.
8. Wear purple on odd numbered days, blue on even.
9. Drink four tablespoons of wine from a baby bottle every Tuesday after sundown.
10. Glue a tampon to your doorbell.

*Note: Please consult your doctor first.

"We still wanted to adopt. That was our plan: we'll have two and we'll adopt one. Anyway we didn't have children. We tried and that was tough. But the moment Oscar arrived, it just felt like he was always meant to come that way. I forget he's adopted; he's just my son."
~Actor Hugh Jackman

#74 The Fertility Diet Doesn't Work

Introducing the next NY Times bestseller, *The Fertility Diet Does Not Work* by Dr. Infertile Naomi. You have read all the books about fertility and diet, but you still aren't pregnant. Does a diet really boost your chances of getting pregnant? The experts say it does but the real experts (the infertiles) know the truth.

This fertility diet says:

Eat dark greens. You once ate spinach and broccoli everyday during your ovulation cycle. How did that work out for you? Better alternative: Green M&Ms and a glass of green beer during Saint Patrick's Day.

Drink Raspberry Leaf Tea. You once let this tea steep for twenty-four hours and drank it cold. Mmmm. It was gross. Better alternative: Raspberry chocolate layer cake. It may not increase your infertility but it sure tastes good.

No alcohol. You don't drink during your cycle but when you know you're not pregnant, watch out pubs! Better alternative: Veal with wine sauce, tiramisu, and a plate of cookies with Baileys poured directly on the biscuits.

Limit your caffeine. You love your coffee in the morning and have switched to decaf. But during your period, you would pour the caffeine directly into your veins, if you could. Better alternative: Drink caffeinated coffee. It just tastes better.

Have more calcium. Studies say that 1,000 milligrams of calcium may improve his sperm count. Better alternative: You know what else will improve his sperm count? Whip cream and chocolate sauce during baby-making sex. Face it, the fertility diet might not work. So let your uterus enjoy a morning coffee with a nice liquor.

#75 How to Avoid Getting Pregnant

How to AVOID getting pregnant (because these fertility tips don't seem to work):

- Make love often during your fertile period.
- Monitor your ovulation by charting your temperature or looking at your cervical fluid.
- Lay down for thirty minutes and do not urinate after intercourse.
- Try powerful fertility drugs and injections.
- Try costly fertility procedures that promise to make you pregnant.
- Reduce your caffeine and alcohol intake.
- Read books on conception and how to get pregnant.
- Avoid vaginal sprays and scented tampons that could kill sperm.
- Make sure your partner avoids hot tubs and biking.
- Exercise and eat healthy.

Congratulations! If you follow all of these tips, you will surely NOT get pregnant. *Disclaimer: Teenage girls and fertile women, do not follow this advice.

#76 Keeping Yourself Occupied in the Fertility Waiting Room

The awkward fertility clinic waiting room can be so quiet that sometimes you just want to break the silence. Whether it's your first fertility appointment (or your hundredth visit), here are some great tips on how to occupy yourself in the waiting room:

1. Snack on an egg.
2. Leave your partner's sperm cup near the magazines.
3. Sing an inspiring song, loudly.
4. Ask the receptionist if they have any sexy videos. It gets your guy going.
5. Accompany your guy to the special room and turn up the volume to a Bette Midler song.
6. Drink some apple juice from a urine sample cup.
7. Put a pillow under your shirt and then waddle around the waiting room.

8. Stick a basal thermometer in your behind and ask someone to check the temperature.
9. Wear a t-shirt that says, 'I'm with an infertile.'
10 Wear a t-shirt that says, 'I did IVF and all I got was this lousy t-shirt.'

#77 The ABCs of Infertility

A – Azoospermia (Help! You have no sperm!)
B – Being Barren
C – Cervical mucus (Your favorite type of mucus!)
D – Donor eggs (Whose your daddy?)
E – Eggs (Do not hard boil or scramble)
F – Failed IUI, failed IVF, failed cycle, F word.
G – Getting pregnant naturally (Tell us your secret!)
H – Hold onto hope
I – In vitro fertilization me
J – Jiggly breasts (Early pregnancy symptom?)
K – Kegel exercises (No need to hit the gym!)
L – Loopy for Lupron
M – Male factor infertility is awesome
N – Negative pregnancy tests (Save your money. Those tests are always negative!)
O – OMG! Ovulation predictor kits
P – PCOS and having your period rocks
Q – Quack (A.k.a your fertility doctor)
R – Rip roaring baby-making sex! (Not as fun as it sounds)
S – Semen analysis cup (Do not drink!)
T – Two week wait (It's definitely not worth the wait!)
U – Urology appointment (Help us, Doctor Balls!)
V – Varicocele veins (Stop heating up that sperm!)
W – When are you going to get pregnant? (World's best question)
X – X-ray that scrotum
Y – Yes we can! (You will get pregnant!)
Z – Zygote (where are you?)

#78 Your Suffer From Infertility Amnesia

Definition of Infertility Amnesia: Referring to an infertile woman who is consumed by her quest to get pregnant that she forgets how lucky and blessed she is in her daily life. A statement meaning to obsess about infertility and disregard everyday joys and happiness. The action of crying and feeling depressed about infertility and forgetting how to laugh and smile.

The good news is there is a cure for this ailment! You have every right to feel how you feel about your situation BUT you can still remember to enjoy life and think about all the other wonderful gifts you already have. It's like you forget about your amazing family, health, friends, and home. Don't suffer from Infertility Amnesia. Don't forget to feel grateful for just being alive.

"The one true hurdle I've faced in life is that I have a broken belly. After years of trying to get pregnant, exploring the range of fertility treatments, all unsuccessful, our journey led us to gestational surrogacy: We make a baby cake and bake it in another woman's oven." ~Actress Elizabeth Banks

#79 Hostile Cervical Mucus

I HATE YOU, SPERM! GO AWAY, CERVIX! LEAVE ME ALONE, UTERUS!

There is nice, friendly and helpful cervical mucus and then there is its moody teenage rival, hostile cervical mucus. The only bodily liquid of its kind that hates everyone and everything. It's not just mean and angry, this cervical mucus is downright hostile, killing anything that gets in its way. You would much rather have hostile saliva, angry snot or moody urine but no, they are all quite friendly and accommodating. They always do their jobs with grace and enthusiasm. You are just one of the lucky ones who happens to have hostile vaginal discharge that likes to kill sperm. No wonder you can't get pregnant. You have World War 3 vaginal discharge. Help! Soldier down. Soldier down.

#80 The Flush and Ring

You take the telephone to the toilet. Your entire day revolves around that important phone call from your fertility nurse. When is she going to call? Why hasn't she phoned yet? Maybe you should call the office. You wait for that call (sometimes all day) to hear the news – your blood work looks great, your embryos are multiplying, the doctor can fit you in tomorrow, your pregnancy test results are in. During the day, you will double check to make sure the phone doesn't have a busy signal, that your answering machine is working and you'll hang up on anyone who isn't your RE (including your own mother).

Waiting all day for that phone call requires drastic measures to be taken. That phone MUST accompany you at all times. If you're sitting on the toilet, enjoying a magazine, chances are the phone is right next to you. Should the phone actually ring, the nurse might hear a slight strain in your voice, delightful gassy background noises and the sound of a flush. Well, at least they called you back.

#81 New Year's Resolution, Infertile Style

It's another New Year's Eve, and you hoped and prayed that this year you would have a baby or at least be pregnant. Instead, you plan to ring in the New Year with a bag of potato chips and a bottle of vodka, for two. But who would want to have a boring last year's pregnancy anyways? Yawn. Snore. Last year, there was a recession, diseases and natural disasters. Who could be pregnant during such negativity anyways? This year will be filled with renewed hope and strength that you are stronger and can get through anything. This coming year brings better looking babies, smarter children and toddlers that will change the world. This year is YOUR year!

Your New Year's Resolutions:

- To cry and obsess about infertility MORE often.
- To buy toilet paper in bulk so you can inspect the TP more frequently without worrying about running out.
- Be environmentally conscious. Re-use pregnancy tests for other uses including donating them to the arts and craft department at your local schools or giving them to a less fortune knocked
up teenager.

Crying about infertility is so last year. Happy New Year! It's a beginning of a new year of hope.

#82 The Chemical Pregnancy Tease

The chemical pregnancy heartache. Another special moment in infertility. A chemical pregnancy, meaning a very early miscarriage, where a positive pregnancy result was detected before her period was due but results in a negative pregnancy test following a period-like bleed.

You were almost there! You had a positive pregnancy test in your hand and something special in your belly. You were just about to throw away your membership to the infertile club and join the fertile pregnancy club. You and your husband got to celebrate the pregnancy for about fifteen minutes when you started to spot. Then you bleed. This doesn't seem right. Take another pregnancy test. Still positive one day and then negative the next. Well, this is confusing. Are you pregnant or aren't you? You were so close, and now the moment is gone, leaving a familiar ache in your chest. You wish you could just put a plug down there to stop the bleeding or perhaps some embryo super glue to stick it back in. You will cry for awhile and hurt for a little longer but then you get up, dry your tears, and learn to smile again.

Bloody hell, infertility! Can't we just get Knocked Up like Katherine Heigl did in that movie or have sex only one time like teenagers do?

#83 The 'I Should Be Pregnant Now' Moment

You've had a lot of special moments during your infertility journey.
The *'This time next year I will be pregnant'* moment.
The *'I can't believe IVF didn't work'* moment.
The *'All my friends are pregnant but me'* moment.

To name just a few… But the 'I SHOULD BE PREGNANT RIGHT NOW' moment is extra fun. You did the fertility treatment and you were so sure that this one was going to work. During the two week wait, you fantasized how you would tell your parents and dreamed about your baby's due date. Then, the negative pregnancy test happens and your fantasies disappear faster than your cervical mucus. You are now left with the 'I should be pregnant right now' moment which includes other special moments like:

- Seeing a pregnant woman and thinking, that should be me!
- Thinking that your six week ultrasound would be next week.
- Knowing that you have to pay for ANOTHER round of treatment.
- Stopping doing your 'I could be pregnant' fake pregnancy waddle.

Now it's your *'I need a strong drink'* moment. Someone grab a drink or two or eight. It's infertility happy hour.

"When you come to the end of your rope, tie a knot and hang on."
~Franklin D. Roosevelt

#84 Hold Onto hope

When you're at the end of your infertile rope, you just cannot cope and (want to smoke dope), hold onto hope. If you just want to mope and overeat cantaloupe, still hold onto hope. When your body says "nope," and your mind says "can't cope," and your tubes can't fallop and you can't remember the last time you used soap, and your heart wants to mope and you Facebook Friended The Pope and your bad breath wants Scope and you want to find a fertile to elope, just say NOPE. You will cope, you won't elope and you will find your HOPE. Tie a knot in your rope and hold tight to hope.

#85 Crying Hysterically Burns Calories

Thinking about going to the gym to lose weight? Think again because infertiles have adopted the 'crying hysterically to burn calories' diet! According to some (unreliable) websites, crying hysterically may actually help you burn calories! Wow. Another great reason to love infertility! Forget those squats, you might be able to burn the same amount of calories simply by looking at a negative pregnancy test and crying for hours!
How does the diet work? It's simple.

Step 1: Commit to crying at least twice an hour, four days a week. 10 CALORIES

Step 2: To maximize calories, flail your arms in a circular and hysterical motion; throw yourself on the ground and blow your nose frequently to burn extra calories. 15 CALORIES.

Step 3: Make sure to breathe. Hyperventilating during emotional breakdowns will increase your heart rate. 10 CALORIES.

Step 4: Release all bodily fluids in excess to help burn excess pounds. Try having severe runny nose and big tears. 30 CALORIES.

Step 5: Keep it simple. Yelling and throwing negative pregnancy tests will exercise muscle tone. 30 CALORIES.

Step 6: Walk to the bathroom and check the toilet paper at least twenty times per day. 25 CALORIES.

Step 7: Make healthier food selections like crying in the organic section of the grocery store and throwing fruits, vegetables, whole grain cereals and low-fat products. 30 CALORIES.

Step 8: Avoid throwing foods that are high in fat and sugar. 5 CALORIES.

Step 9: Have a variety of emotional breakdowns in your nutritional plan. Try crying during a yoga or cardio class. 40 CALORIES.

Step 10: Have realistic goals. Don't just toss your negative pregnancy stick in the garbage. Try to rip it in half or hurl it through a glass window. 40 CALORIES.

The 'crying hysterically to burn calories' diet really works! Just ask any fertility-medicated and
bloated infertile.

#86 Mommy Friends Talk About Poop

Have you ever gotten together with your mommy friends and felt really left out of the conversation because you didn't have a baby? It's a Saturday afternoon and you are at your mommy friend's house where everyone has a baby but you. The conversation quickly turns into mommy talk. *"Oh my goodness, little Sandy had the biggest poop last night. Is a mustard color bowel movement normal?"* *"Little Penny hasn't pooped in four whole days! Should I take her to the pediatrician?"*

In mommyland, talking about baby poop and diarrhea is completely normal but you have nothing to contribute to the conversation unless you talk about your own bowel movements. *"Hey, I just made a huge dump this morning. It was brown."* But no one wants to hear about that. Mommies want to talk to other mommies and when there is a non-mommy in the room, you might as well be invisible. You can't provide advice about her breastfeeding issue and you have no idea what the Goo-Goo Sleep Training Method is. It's like if you opened your mouth and talked about the color and consistency of your own cervical mucus or your latest IUI. *"My cervical mucus was simply splendid this month,"* you would say (as you sip your glass of wine). *"It's consistency and texture was just divine!"*

Instead, you smile politely, nodding your head every once and awhile while inside you feel like someone is ripping a piece of your heart. And the only way to cope with a broken heart is to overeat and drink as soon as you get home. Just try to erase the image of baby Mitzy's yellow and green stained diaper from your memory.

#87 The Fertility Frappuccino

Dear Starbucks Customer Service,

You should really offer your female customers a Menstrual Cycle Day, half-priced Frappuccino. This will help decrease our anger and make us feel just a tiny bit better as we have an emotional breakdown inside your bathroom. You can call it the Bitchin' Grande, Extra Caffeinated, Extra Mocha, My Period Just Arrived, High Fat, Whipped and Spiked Frappuccino. Listed below, I have also included some other Frappuccino suggestions for your coffee menu.

Frappuccino Suggestions

I Just Peed on a Negative Pregnancy Test Frappuccino
Drizzled with some 'why the hell did I waste money on another pregnancy stick' syrup; combined with extra caffeinated (non-decaf) coffee, fresh extra fat milk; blended with ice and heartache, and deliciously topped with whipped cream and a swirl of f--k this!

The Male Factor Infertility Frappuccino
A unique combination of multi-vitamins including Vitamin E and Zinc; topped with 'you better stay away from that hot tub' syrup; a touch of coffee and fresh (non-soy) milk; blended with extra ice (no overheating!) and sprinkled with regular exercise and a healthy weight. Drink no more than every other day.

The Relax and It Will Happen Frappuccino
A stress-free blend of 'your fertility advice sucks' syrup; sprinkled with 'I went on vacation and didn't come back pregnant' topping; blended with some decadent 'I stopped thinking about it and it didn't happen' cookie crumble. Extra caffeinated, please.

The Failed IVF Frappuccino
A painful blend of a negative beta mixed with 'I just paid $10,000 for my period' sauce; drizzled with 'I still have leftover fertility drugs in

my refrigerator' and spiked with alcohol. This Frappuccino should be free of charge considering you have no money left.

The Kickin' Infertility Ass Frappuccino
A decadent blend of optimism and perseverance; combined with determination and a little acupuncture; sprinkled with everlasting hope, baby dust and lots of chocolate.

#88 Why Am I Not Pregnant Yet

Why am I not pregnant yet? I ask. I plead. I beg,
why won't Mr. Sperm just fertilize my egg?

It feels like everyone is pregnant, everyone but us,
please let us jump on board the crowded fertile bus.

Baby bumps are everywhere! Please just grant our wish,
even our goldfish, Patches, is expecting a baby fish!

Celebrities seem to sport a bump and a pregnant glow,
while I get bloated from fertility meds and curse my Aunty Flow.

We have tried EVERYTHING from doctors to special tea,
every month, we plant our seed so fertilize my tree!

And then we have to wait and wait to get our special sign,
but still a negative pregnancy test flashes just one line.

I can't wait to be a mom, it will fill my life with roses,
bring on the dirty diapers, puke and runny noses!

Our hearts are filled with anguish and our throats just have a lump,
we just want our miracle baby and that special baby bump.

But one day it will be our turn, I really do believe,
our miracle will happen and then I will conceive.

Until then, we will save our tears and just learn how to cope,
we will still enjoy our lives while holding onto hope.

"When your dreams turn to dust, vacuum." ~unknown

#89 Count the Pregnant Women

There's one… There's one… There's one… Oh wait. She's just fat. Thank goodness. Every time you leave the house, it feels like every single pregnant woman on earth decides to walk past you. Every place you turn, someone's pregnant, sporting a baby bump, pushing a stroller or even worse, pushing a stroller and holding onto a toddler's hand. How come she gets two babies when you can't even get one? A fun game to play is, 'count the pregnant women.' Betcha can't count just one! There's one. There's one. Hey, there's another! It's a super fun game to play because you can play it anywhere, from a baby shower or every single time you leave your house! Walking down the street – there's a bump. Going to the grocery story – there's a fertile in the pickle aisle. At the gym – hey look, it's pregnancy fit hour. Neat-o!

Don't you wish that you could just carry a sign that read, 'I'm feeling lonely. Any other infertile in the crowd? If so, wave your ovulation stick.' But if you want to know if there are any other infertile's out there, just look at her eyes. She will be staring at a pregnant belly. Damn. It's a full time job being this bitter and jealous all of the time.

#90 You are the Designated Infertile Driver

Why does being infertile suddenly make you the designated driver? And we're not talking about drinking and driving. For some reason, you are always responsible for driving someone home, doing a quick favor or running an errand simply because you don't have kids. Your fertile sibling gets out of all errands and responsibilities simply because she/he is a parent. You get this: *"Can you drive Aunt Gertie home tonight? I know your sister lives in the same apartment building and you live on the other side of town, but your sister has the baby."* And sometimes you get this: *"Don't worry,* (insert your name here), *will bring all the side dishes for dinner. I would have asked* (insert fertile sibling name) *but she has the baby."* And sometimes this happens: *"Can you help with the dishes tonight. I would ask* (insert fertile sibling name) *but she's pregnant and she needs to rest."* (Ummm. You've just had embryos removed from your uterus but sure thing, you can scrub the kitchen floor).

You are the designated infertile driver. Just remember, an IUI and a DUI are not the same things so drive responsibly.

#91 Phoning Your Mommy Friend

RING. RING.

You: *"Hi (fertile friend). Just calling to say hello."*

Mommy Friend: *"Nice to hear from y— JESSICA, GET OFF THE SOFA!— How are things with you and—TOMMY, DO YOU HAVE A POOPIE DIAPER AGAIN? — Sorry about that, what were you saying — ONE MORE SCREAM AND YOU'RE SITTING IN THE CORNER, YOUNG LADY."*

Remember when you use to call your friend (pre-child) and you could actually have a conversation with her without interruptions? Now, you are reluctant to phone her because you know she will be chatting with both you and her kiddies at the same time. You can't really blame her. But you would have liked to talk to your friend without having to listen to her sing a Sesame Street song. It's hard to chat about your latest fertility treatment when she's multi-tasking with a baby suckling on her nipple and changing a diaper with her free hand.

"Do you want me to call back at a better time?" you ask her politely. *"Oh no,"* she says.

"I'm free to chat now–SALLIE-SUE, IF YOU DON'T GET OFF THAT KITCHEN TABLE—..." Is it impolite if you ask your mommy friend to lock her children in another room?

"Sorry about that," mommy friend says. *"Now, what were you saying about your lack of cervical mucu—- MARTHA, I'M GOING TO COUNT TO THREE —ONE, TWO..."*

So long mommy friend. CLICK.

#92 Bad Fertility Advice

Possibly the worst advice you can ever give an infertile is 'just relax and it will happen.' Are you KIDDING us? The only thing that's relaxed right now is his sperm because they don't seem to be swimming. Please tell us, Great Aunt Jean, when should I relax?

- After I've just spent $10,000 on fertility treatments?
- When I'm injecting fertility needles into my ass?
- When I'm swallowing medications to make me more hormonal?
- When I'm wondering if I'm going to live the rest of my life childless and with cats?
- When I'm doing acupuncture and sticking tiny needles into my face and stomach?
- When I'm having timed intercourse and then sticking pillows under my butt?
- When I'm sticking a thermometer into my mouth each morning to chart my temperature?
- When I have to wake up before 4am to drive to my early morning blood and ultrasound appointment?
- When my RE is sticking an odd looking transvaginal wand into my lady parts?
- When I'm inserting vaginal suppositories in a public bathroom?
- Thanks so much for the advise, auntie, but I'll pass.

#93 Good Morning, Lady Parts!

Remember the good old days when you had a pap smear and only ONE doctor looked into your lady parts? Those were the days. During your fertility journey, you now have an assortment of doctors, interns, nurses, ultrasound technicians examining your lower region. It's like a party down there.

As if going for fertility treatments wasn't awkward enough. Why must everyone in your city get to examine your lady parts on a daily basis? And don't expect the doctor to even know your name. You are probably just known as Vagina Number 3004.

The embryo transfer is no better, except that even more strangers are in the room, enjoying the view. *"Hey, isn't that Doogie Howser over there?" "Oh look, even the secretary came by for the show!" "Hey, isn't that your Great Aunt Agnes? I'm glad she could make it."* In some clinics, they also shine a bright light directly into your lady parts. Who is the star of the show now? It feels like a broadway musical starring your vagina. But you would let the entire cast of the Vagina Monologues come into your ultrasound appointment if it meant it would get you pregnant.

- Number of people that have seen your lady parts during your fertility appointments: 10-20

- Number of interns that have enjoyed your transvaginal wand show: 15-20
- Getting pregnant from a fertility treatments: Priceless

"Don't be discouraged. It's often the last key in the bunch that opens the lock." ~unknown

#94 What to Expect When You're Not Expecting

When you're not expecting, you'll find many books to tell you how to get pregnant. You know which books they are because most of them are currently sitting on your nightstand. Perhaps you've read *Six Easy Steps to Increase your Fertility; The IVF Baby; Conquering Infertility in Three Days;* and *Taking Charge of your Cervical Mucus,* to name just a few. Well, you've taken charge of your fertility and where the fertile has it gotten you? Twenty thousand dollars poorer, twenty pounds heavier and over twenty failed cycles. When it comes to fertility books, you have read them all. It's like book publishers can sense your infertile desperation and they keep publishing more and more books on the subject.

Here are some more realistic fertility books:

What to Expect after you've peed on a stick and you're not sure if you really see a second line or it's your imagination.

What to Expect when you've been waiting all day for the fertility doctor to call you back.

What to Expect after you've had baby-making sex, not because you wanted to, but because it was ovulation time.

What to Expect when cousin Martha gets pregnant on her first try.

What to Expect when you have way too much PCOS-related facial hair.

What to Expect after you've been inseminated by a twenty year old fertility intern named Teresa.

What to Expect when your Facebook friends happily post their ultrasound photos and you want to shoot yourself.

What to Expect after you've just eaten a container of ice cream following a BFN.

What to Expect when you're at a baby shower sobbing in the guest of honor's bathroom.

What to Expect when you have to give yourself a fertility injection during cousin Emma's wedding.

What to Expect when you feel hopeless but you know you will never give up HOPE.

#95 Dear Fertility Santa

Dear Fertility Santa,

How are you? Mrs. Claus treating you well? Santa, I have been a very good girl this year. I have taken my folic acid on a daily basis (minus last month when I said 'screw you, folic acid' during a very bad menstrual period). I have stuck a thermometer in my mouth every single morning to chart my temperature (and have only cheated twice by taking my temperature after my shower). Even last week when we went out for dinner, I didn't look at the toilet paper once when I went to the bathroom at Mork's Fine Steakhouse. Santa, I was a very good girl when my husband had a three day business trip during my peak ovulation period. I only overacted a little bit by begging him to stay home, then crying hysterically over a bowl of mint chip ice cream.

Then, there was the time when I acted super strong after my failed cycle and then cried only a little in front of a Walmart cashier. I was even really good after my friend, Bessie-Sue, posted all her pregnancy belly photos on Facebook (if you refer to photo number four hundred in an album called, My Six Month Belly Picture), you will even see that I nicely commented, *"Hey Bessie-Sue, your belly looks great!"* That's pretty darn nice, if you ask me.

Santa, my husband has also been a very good boy. He went for his semen analysis test without putting up a fuss. He didn't get mad at me when I made him watch a documentary called, '*I have Limited Sperm, Now What*?' and he even took a stack of vitamins to increase his sperm count. Santa, there was also the time when his sister got pregnant with her third accidental baby and he spared telling me until we got home. I'd say that this year, we have both been pretty darn good. Please fill our stockings with baby dust and fill our Christmas tree with light and hope and determination. Please bring us strength and optimism and fill our hearts with positive thoughts in the new year.

With Love, Infertile in the City

#96 Your Facebook Friend's Profile is an Avocado

Your pregnant Facebook friend, Sally, is a real fruit. Each week fertile Sally updates her
Facebook profile picture with a fruit-related photo to correspond to her pregnancy.

Week 12: Sally's profile photo says that her baby is the size of a lemon!
Week 14: Sally's baby is the size of a red delicious apple!
Week 15: Sally's baby is an orange!

Last night, you innocently (purposely) checked your Facebook account to see that Sally had changed her profile picture to an avocado. Either Sally became a big fan of avocados or she is sixteen weeks pregnant. Her second baby fruit in two years. Sigh.

But just because Sally's baby daddy thinks that Sally is the apple of his eye and stuck his banana into her pear only one time, and made a little snow pea, doesn't mean she has to go bananas and make a whole fruit salad announcement on Facebook. Sally, you're a real peach. Orange you glad you're an infertile?

#97 Infertility jokes

Infertility is no joke. There is nothing funny about transvaginal wands; having a fertility doctor looking at your lower region at 7:00 in the morning or lying to your boss when you arrive late to work because you were having eggs surgically removed from your ovaries. Infertility is no laughing matter, unless you are telling infertility jokes! Enjoy some of these jokes courtesy of the awesome women and men on the 999 Reasons to Laugh at Infertility blog and Facebook pages!

- At 8:50 PM, an infertile walks into a bar. Bartender says, "can I get you a shot?" Infertile says, "not for another 10 minutes, but I'll take a margarita while I wait."

- You know you are trying to get pregnant when...Someone asks you today's date and you reply "Day 21."

- How does an RE like his eggs? Over 20mm!

- Why did the woman cross the road? Because there was a fertility clinic on the other side.

- Why does it take 50 million sperm to fertilize one egg? Because they won't ask for directions either!

"When it's dark enough, you can see the stars." ~Ralph Waldo Emerson

#98 Saint Patrick's Day, Infertile Style

During infertility, you tend to hate all holidays. A baby-less Christmas was not fun. Your birthday was the worst. Mother's/Father's Day made you turn to drinking and even International Asparagus Day made you a little teary eyed. But it's almost Saint Patrick's Day. The day where pregnant women are banned from all bars and you can wallow in your sorrows by drinking green beer!

Here are some tips on how to spend Saint Patrick's Day, Infertile Style!

1. Wear a pair of good luck green underwear to your transvaginal appointment.
2. Start your day with Lucky Charms cereal to give you some luck.
3. Ask your fertility doctor to paint your fertilized embryos green.
4. Find a leprechaun to rub your belly.
5. Ask your partner to dress like a leprechaun and get busy.
6. Pour some green food coloring into your husband's semen analysis cup.
7. Paint your face green and pretend that you have morning sickness.
8. Find a four leaf clover and ask your RE to insert it directly into your uterus.

#99 Infertility Makes You Weird

Remember the good old days when you had no idea what cervical mucus was; you didn't chart your temperature first thing in the morning; and you didn't have an emotional breakdown if your husband was unavailable during your peak ovulation period. Infertility has made you weird.

Remember the days when you used birth control pills so you wouldn't get pregnant? When your older cousin announced her pregnancy and you didn't burst into tears? When you would walk past a pregnant woman without glaring and feeling jealous of her baby bump? Your life has now changed. Oh, how it has changed.

You now know your husband's exact sperm count and the rate of his motility (*"But doctor, his count was one million during our last appointment and his motility has gone up ten percent"*). You now have fertility medication in your refrigerator, right next to the milk and last night's leftover quiche (Dinner time! Tonight we're having meatloaf or Progesterone). You google all your fake pregnancy symptoms including (and not limited to), *I have a cold. Am I pregnant? I have a strange twitches on my left side. Am I pregnant? My right breast feels more swollen than my left. Am I pregnant already?* Infertility has made your weird. But it's not your fault. Blame infertility.

Infertile Naomi's Pregnancy Tips

I am not a pregnancy expert. If I were, I would have conceived the first month we tried and had my own television reality show called, 'I Coughed and got Pregnant.' I was able to finally conceive through the magic of IVF, a fertility clinic, medication, and a kick ass petri dish. None the less, my blog readers often ask about my successful IVF, so here are my personal tips. Please always consult your doctor about your individual situation.

Acupuncture for Fertility
During my successful IVF (fresh) cycle, I did fertility acupuncture one hour before my transfer and immediately following. Acupuncture is supposed to improve blood flow to the uterine arteries and allow the uterus to relax.

What the Prolactin?!
Our fertility issue was diagnosed as male factor infertility (*Honey, you need more sperm*). During our successful IVF cycle, my doctor thought that my prolactin levels were a tiny bit elevated and put me on medication to lower it. I remained on this medication until I was six weeks pregnant.

The Fertility Diet
During my years trying to conceive, I exercised and tried to eat a balance diet, with multi-vitamins and limited caffeine. However, when I got my period, I participated in the 'Screw You Infertility' Diet which included, delicious caffeinated beverages and alcohol. During my successful cycle, I did drink both caffeinated and decaf coffee and still enjoyed the occasional sweet treat. Basically, I ate normally.

Embryos Don't Like Heat
My fertility doctor told me that embryos don't like the heat. They advised me not to use a car seat warmer and stay away from hot baths. My husband was also banned from hot tubs and bicycling. Apparently, sperm doesn't like the heat either.

Watch America Idol
I watched a lot of television during my two week wait. I didn't 'just relax' but I did enjoy my time, just being good to myself. I also watched an insane amount of American Idol and I'm pretty sure my embryos got bored of listening to the show and decided to implant.

Positive Thoughts
Staying positive during the long road to parenthood is difficult. I decided that during every medicated cycle, I would be as positive as possible. During my successful IVF cycle, I told myself (and my uterus, if she was listening) everyday, that I was pregnant. I sent positive thoughts to my body and even said them aloud (although strangers on the street did think I was strange)! Whether positive thinking worked or not, I felt better, stronger and happier.

Whatever your own personal road to parenthood, remember to stay positive and keep smiling. From infertility, comes strength.

For more infertile humor and support, please check out the blog!

999 Reasons to Laugh at Infertility Blog: www.999reasonstolaugh.com
Twitter: @InfertileNaomi
999 Reasons on Facebook

INSPIRATIONAL QUOTES

"It does not matter how slowly you go so long as you do not stop." ~Confucius

"Our greatest glory is not in never failing, but in rising up every time we fail." ~Ralph Waldo Emerson

"When you feel like giving up, remember why you held on for so long in the first place." ~Unknown

"When the world says, "Give up," Hope whispers, 'Try it one more time." ~Unknown

"Courage is going from failure to failure without losing enthusiasm." ~Winston Churchill

"A bend in the road is not the end of the road...unless you fail to make the turn." ~Unknown

"The difficulties of life are intended to make us better, not bitter." ~Unknown

"All it takes is one bloom of hope to make a spiritual garden." ~Tern Guillemets

"When life takes the wind out of your sails, it is to test you at the oars." ~Robert Brault

"Failure is the condiment that gives life its flavor." ~Truman Capote

"Once you choose hope, anything's possible." ~Christopher Reeve

"There is no telling how many miles you have to run while chasing a dream." ~Unknown

"I may not be there yet, but I am closer than I was yesterday." ~Unknown

"I can't imagine the direction of the wind, but I can adjust my sails to always reach my destination." ~Jimmy Dean

"There are only two ways to live your life. One is as though nothing is a miracle. The other is as though everything is a miracle." ~Albert Einstein

"If opportunity doesn't knock, build a door." ~Milton Berle

Printed in Great Britain
by Amazon